AUTOIMMUNITY

THE MEDICAL PERSPECTIVES SERIES

Editors:

Andrew P. Read *Department of Medical Genetics, University of Manchester, St Mary's Hospital, Hathersage Road, Manchester M13 0JH, U.K.*

Terence Brown *Department of Biochemistry and Applied Molecular Biology, UMIST, Manchester M60 1QD, U.K.*

Oncogenes and Tumor Suppressor Genes

Cytokines

The Human Genome

Autoimmunity

Genetic Engineering (due 1992)

Asthma (due early 1993)

AUTOIMMUNITY

W. Ollier and D.P.M. Symmons
*ARC Epidemiology Research Unit, Medical School,
University of Manchester, Oxford Road,
Manchester M13 9PT, U.K.*

© BIOS Scientific Publishers Limited, 1992

First published in the United Kingdom 1992 by
BIOS Scientific Publishers Limited,
St Thomas House, Becket Street, Oxford OX1 1SJ.

A CIP catalogue record for this book is available from the British Library.

ISBN 1 872 748 50 3

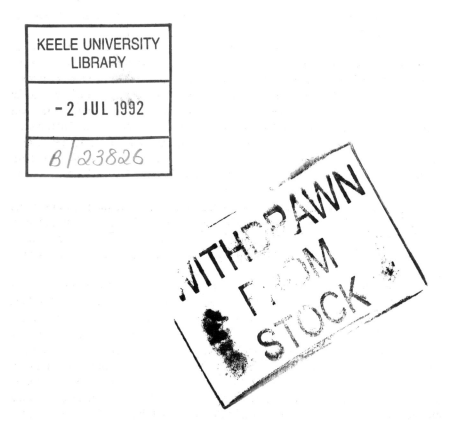

Typeset by Enset Photosetting Limited, Bath, U.K.
Printed by Information Press Ltd, Oxford, U.K.

PREFACE

In 1899 Paul Ehrlich coined the term 'horror autotoxicus' to describe the potential situation in which the immune system of the body might turn against itself. In his description the concept of autoimmunity was born. Since that time it has been recognized that many diseases have an autoimmune etiology. These diseases are very diverse in their clinical manifestations. Almost every system and organ of the body may be attacked by an autoimmune process – and so all clinicians have an interest in the phenomenon.

The attempt to understand the mechanisms whereby the normal self-tolerance of the immune system may break down has drawn in scientists from many fields. As each of these areas of basic science advances so does the understanding of autoimmunity. It is clear that susceptibility to many autoimmune diseases has a genetic basis. As the molecular biologist and geneticist unravel the mystery of gene structure, the exact epitopes responsible for disease susceptibility are being identified. Similarly, understanding of the normal roles of all the cells and mediators in the immune system is enabling breaches in the defense, which may lead to autoimmunity, to be identified. All the theories developed must be compatible with the observed clinical patterns of the diseases both within individuals and within populations.

This book originates from an Epidemiology Research Unit and is written by an immunologist and a clinician/epidemiologist. We hope it will be of interest to clinical medical students, non-specialists working in medicine, and also other postgraduate scientists encountering autoimmune diseases for the first time but with little knowledge of clinical medicine.

The book begins by looking at the components and role of the normal immune system. The phenomenon of self-tolerance and its development is described and the concept of autoimmunity occurring as a result of the breakdown of self-tolerance is introduced. In the second chapter the genetic susceptibility to autoimmune disease is examined. Chapter 3 looks at the definition and characterization of auto-antigens. Chapter 4 examines the consequences of autoimmunity at the cellular and humoral level. It includes a section on methods of measuring auto-antibodies. Having started at the level of the gene and progressed to that of the cell, the book then looks at the clinical consequences of autoimmunity. Multi-system autoimmune disease and organ-specific diseases are described. Treatment options are explored and there is a section on experimental immunomodulation. Finally the book looks at the prognosis of autoimmunity and the problem of malignant complications.

We have endeavored to provide as current a view as possible but this is a constantly changing field and every week the journals publish more articles which contribute to our understanding of autoimmunity. Rather than provide long and overpowering lists of references for each chapter we have suggested a number of well-referenced review articles and textbooks which will enable the reader to gain more detailed information. A brief glossary of terms is also provided to help the reader.

We should like to thank Irene Smith for her patience in typing the manuscript and preparing the line drawings.

W.Ollier

D.P.M.Symmons

CONTENTS

ABBREVIATIONS

α1-AT	alpha 1 anti-trypsin
AChR	acetylcholine receptor
ACTH	adrenocorticotrophic hormone
AD	autoimmune disease
ADCC	antibody-dependent cellular cytotoxicity
AIDS	acquired immune deficiency syndrome
AIHA	autoimmune hemolytic anemia
AMA	antimitochondrial antibody
ANA	antinuclear antibody
APC	antigen presenting cell
Asn	asparagine
ASO	allele-specific oligonucleotide probes
Asp	aspartic acid
bp	base pair
C	constant region
CAH	chronic active hepatitis
CD	cluster of differentiation
cDNA	complementary DNA
CFA	complete Freund's adjuvant
CREST	calcinosis, Raynaud's, esophageal involvement, sclerodactyly, telangiectasia
CTL	cytotoxic T lymphocyte
D	diversity region
DNA	deoxyribonucleic acid
dNTPs	deoxynucleotide 5'-triphosphates
dsDNA	double-stranded DNA
DZ	dizygotic
EAE	experimental autoimmune encephalomyelitis
EBV	Epstein–Barr virus
ELISA	enzyme-linked immunosorbent assay
ENA	extractable nuclear antigen
FITC	fluorescein isothiocyanate
GM–CSF	granulocyte and monocyte colony stimulating factor
GPC	gastric parietal cell
H-2	H-2 gene complex (mouse MHC)
HIV	human immunodeficiency virus
HLA	human leukocyte antigen
HSP	heat shock protein
IF	intrinsic factor
IFN	interferon
IgA/D/G/E/M	immunoglobulin A/D/G/E/M
IL	interleukin
ITP	idiopathic thrombocytopenic purpura

J	joining region
kd	kilodalton
LAK	lymphocyte-activated killer cells
LFA	lymphocyte functional antigen
LKM	liver and kidney microsomes
LOD	logarithm of the odds
LPS	lipopolysaccharide
LSP	liver-specific protein
MBP	myelin basic protein
MG	myasthenia gravis
MHC	major histocompatibility complex
mRNA	messenger RNA
MS	multiple sclerosis
MSH	melanocyte stimulating hormone
MZ	monozygotic
NK	natural killer
NOD	non-obese diabetic mouse
PA	pernicious anemia
PBC	primary biliary cirrhosis
PCR	polymerase chain reaction
PI	protease inhibitor
PLA2	phospholipase A2
PSS	progressive systemic sclerosis
PTH	parathyroid hormone
RA	rheumatoid arthritis
RANA	rheumatoid arthritis nuclear antigen
RBC	red blood cell
RF	rheumatoid factor
RFLP	restriction fragment length polymorphism
RNA	ribonucleic acid
RNP	ribonuclear protein
S	sedimentary coefficient
SA	superantigen
SLE	systemic lupus erythematosus
SMA	smooth muscle antibody
snRNP	small nuclear ribonuclear protein
SS	Sjögren's Syndrome
TI-DM	Type I-diabetes mellitus
T3	tri-iodothyronine
T4	thyroxine
TCR	T cell receptor
TG	thyroglobulin
Ti	idiotypic T cell receptor
TNF	tumor necrosis factor
TPO	thyroid peroxidase
TRH	thyrotrophin-releasing hormone
tRNA	transfer RNA
TSH	thyroid-stimulating hormone
V	variable region
YAC	yeast artificial chromosome

1
INTRODUCTION

1.1 The role of the immune system

The immune system is the police force of the body. Its prime functions are to protect the body from invading micro-organisms and to provide surveillance against cells which have become malignant. The first line of defense against invasion is non-specific and highly effective. Only when this is breached does the full force of the acquired immune system come into play. Acquired immunity has four important features:

- It is specific – an immune response directed against a particular agent will not recognize or be effective against other agents.

- It is acquired – before exposure to the agent no immunity exists.

- It has memory – once immunity has been induced subsequent rechallenge produces a rapid response.

- It can discriminate between self and non-self. One of the central dogmas of immunity is that the immune system does not react against 'self'. Any agent not present in the body is treated as foreign.

Much applied immunological research has been directed at trying to manipulate these 'truths'. With regard to self–non-self recognition, the transplantation biologist and surgeon would like to convince the immune system that foreign grafts are the same as self and need not be rejected and destroyed. In contrast, the tumor immunologist would like actively to encourage the immune response to regard self-malignant cells as foreign and eliminate them from the body. Nature provides an intriguing exception to the rule of self–non-self recognition in the phenomenon of autoimmunity. In this situation the immune response recognizes and responds to part of the body (an auto-antigen) producing an autoimmune disease (AD).

1.2 The components of the immune system

The immune system is made up of central lymphoid tissue (bone marrow, thymus), secondary lymphoid tissues (spleen, lymph nodes, Peyer's patches in the intestine) and circulating lymphocytes. Lymphoid tissue comprises about 3% of body weight. The lymphoid structures are linked by a system of lymphatics which conduct lymphocytes from the blood, through the tissues and lymph nodes and back into the bloodstream (*Figure 1.1*).

Lymphocytes are the fulcrum of the immune system. Their roles include antigen recognition, the production of various chemical intercellular mediators (cytokines/lymphokines), and synthesis of antibodies. There are two major classes of lymphocyte: B cells (so called because in birds they are derived from the Bursa of Fabricius) and T cells (so called because they are processed by the thymus). There is no precise mammalian equivalent of the Bursa of Fabricius. In man, B cells are derived from the bone marrow. T and B cells have different functional capabilities: B cells can differentiate to become plasma cells and secrete antibodies, whereas T lymphocytes sub-divide into effector and regulatory cells. Effector T cells are responsible for cell-mediated immune reactions, the elimination of virus infections and tumor rejection. Regulatory T cells may either enhance or diminish the responses of B or T lymphocytes.

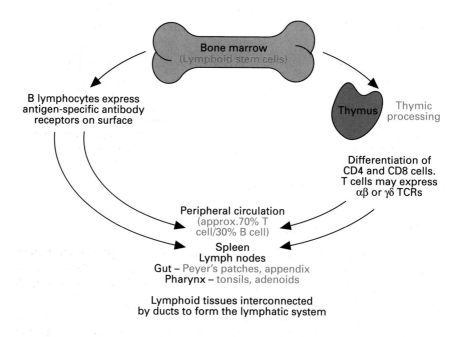

Figure 1.1: *Components of the immune system.*

In order to become a functioning cell, the resting lymphocyte must first be activated. This occurs as a result of antigen recognition. A limited number of antigens can activate B cells directly, but most B cell responses require additional help and co-operation from T cells (*Figure 1.2*). T cell antigens must be presented on the surface of other cells in conjunction with self-determinants of the major histocompatibility complex (MHC) (Section 2.5). The phenomenon of MHC-restriction of T cell function is central to the understanding of autoimmunity.

Class II positive cells such as macrophages, dendritic cells or B
lymphocytes are required to present antigen to αβ T cells

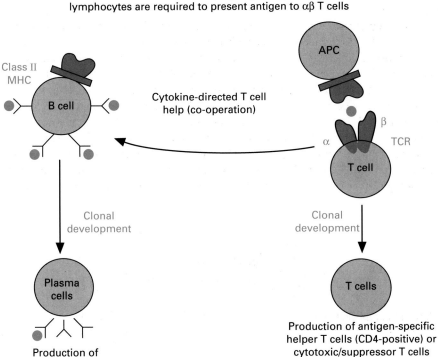

Figure 1.2: *B and T lymphocyte responses.*

1.2.1 B cells and antibodies

The immunological hallmark of B cells is the presence of immunoglobulin on their cell surface. Immunoglobulins are made up of glycosylated disulfide-bridged light and heavy polypeptide chains, each of which is divided into a 'variable' region that binds antigen and a 'constant' region that controls effector functions (*Figure 1.3*).

A single B cell will produce only one specificity of antibody with a uniform binding site. There are five classes of heavy chain – γ, α, μ, δ and ε – giving rise to the five immunoglobulin classes IgG, A, M, D and E. There are four subclasses of IgG and two subclasses of IgA. The heavy chain constant regions associated with the different classes and subclasses of immunoglobulin are termed isotypes. A normal individual would be expected to have all nine isotypic variants in his serum. There are two types of light chain – κ and λ. Each B cell can only produce one type of light chain.

There is also between-individual variation in the structure of immunoglobulins. This variation usually involves one or two amino acids in the constant region of the heavy chains. These changes give rise to what are termed allotypic variants.

The variable regions of light and heavy chains are not variable throughout their whole length and there are a number of 'hypervariable regions'. These regions are intimately involved in the formation of the antigen binding site. As well as recognizing a given antigen, these hypervariable regions may themselves be immunogenic. Indeed,

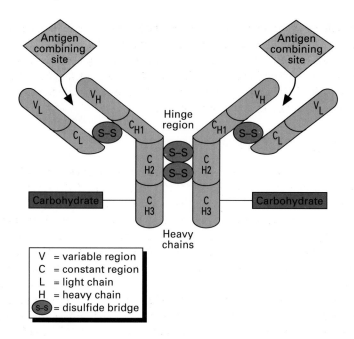

Figure 1.3: *The immunoglobulin molecule..*

there may be more than one part of the hypervariable domain which is antigenic. Each of these sites is termed an idiotype and the antibodies which specifically recognize these sites are termed anti-idiotypic.

Each human haplotype encoding immunoglobulin genes includes approximately 100–200 heavy chain variable genes (V), 100 κ light chain V genes and an unknown number of λ light chain V genes. Early in B cell ontogeny, a functional light chain immunoglobulin gene is generated by rearrangement of one V gene with a separate joining (J) gene segment. For heavy chains, an additional gene segment for diversity (D) couples with the J segment prior to V gene addition. This rearrangement, together with insertional inaccuracies produced during gene recombination and somatic mutations of V region genes, produces an almost limitless repertoire of antigen combining sites which can be 'spliced' with genes for the constant heavy chains of the antibody molecule.

Antibody production. Antibody production, in most cases, is a two-step procedure. First, the antigen concerned must be recognized and bound by immunoglobulin expressed on the surface of B cells. The B cell then requires a 'second signal' in the form of lymphokines produced by helper (CD4-positive) T cells. The T helper cell must recognize both the antigen and the MHC components on the B cell. This B/T cell co-operation is antigen specific.

Having recognized the antigen and received a second T cell signal, the B lymphocyte divides, expanding into a clone of cells producing antibody with exactly the same specificity as that of the cell originally triggered. End cells of this expansion are called plasma cells. They produce and secrete antibody molecules in large quantities. Although the specificity of the antibody never changes, given a suitable lymphokine signal, IgM antibodies can class-switch to IgG.

The regulation of clonal expansion of B cells is not fully understood. One major regulatory system is thought to be the idiotypic network, first suggested by Jerne in 1974 (Section 4.4.3). Failure of regulation can lead to malignant transformation of plasma cells, a condition called malignant myeloma.

1.2.2 T cell sub-sets and the T cell receptor

A variety of specific antigens on the T cell surface have been detected with the help of monoclonal antibodies. This has led to the identification of T cell sub-sets which differ either in function or in their state of activation. A uniform system of nomenclature is now used to distinguish these T cell marker antigens, each of which begins with the initials CD (cluster of differentiation). All peripheral T cells have the antigens CD2, CD3 and CD5. In addition they bear either the CD4 or the CD8 antigen. As well as stimulating antibody production by B cells, CD4-positive T cells also help cytotoxic T cells become functional and macrophages to become activated. The CD8-positive population includes at least two functionally different sub-sets – the effector cytotoxic T cells which can kill virally infected or foreign cells, and suppressor T cells which can regulate the immune response. Presentation of antigen to both CD4 and CD8 T cells is intimately connected with MHC antigen expression. This is discussed more fully in Chapter 2. In the peripheral blood approximately 60% of T cells are CD4-positive and 40% CD8-positive. In the germinal centers of lymph nodes more than 90% of T cells are CD4-positive.

Much work has been done in recent years on characterizing the T cell antigen receptor (TCR). It has much in common with the equivalent receptor on B cells – the immunoglobulin molecule. The T cell receptor consists of the CD3 molecule (which is made up of non-covalently linked polypeptide chains) and Ti (the idiotypic T cell receptor) which is a heterodimer composed of two disulfide-bonded polypeptide chains. Two types of Ti are found: one comprising α and β chains; the other γ and δ chains (Section 2.6.3). Each chain is composed of a variable and a constant region. The variable regions are the products of genes for variable (V), joining (J) and diversity (D) segments for β and δ chains and V and J segments for α and γ chains.

1.2.3 Cytokines

In the late 1960s it was realized that a variety of soluble mediators are produced in the course of an immune response which have widespread effects on lymphocytes and other cells. These mediators were originally called 'lymphokines' and 'monokines' depending on whether they were produced by lymphocytes or monocytes/macrophages. Early studies were hampered by having only semi-purified material to work with which contained mixtures of factors. Later the term 'interleukin' was coined, with each factor being given an identifying number (e.g. IL-1). It has since become clear that many interleukins affect not only leukocytes but also other cell types. The term now favored is 'cytokine'. A cytokine is defined as being a polypeptide mediator which regulates cellular activity (growth, differentiation or function) by binding to a specific receptor. The term does not include mediators released as neurotransmitters nor hormones of the endocrine and neuro-endocrine systems.

As summarized in *Figure 1.4* many cytokines are produced by macrophages and lymphocytes. In addition cytokines are made by other cell types such as fibroblasts and endothelial cells. CD4-positive cells produce a series of cytokines as a consequence of recognizing a peptide–self-MHC class II complex and receiving a second signal (IL-1) from the antigen presenting cell. Cytokines produce a variety of immunological and physiological effects (see *Figure 1.4*). There is an overlap in function between some cytokines. Cytokines also influence the production of other cytokines giving rise to a complex regulatory network. At the center of this network is the helper T cell recognizing antigen.

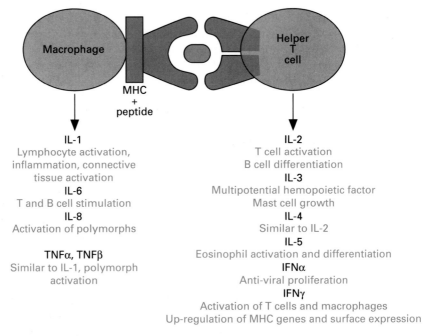

Figure 1.4: *Cytokine production.*

Cytokines produced by helper T cells control the immune response at different levels. IL-2 is a T cell growth factor, IL-3 a mast cell growth factor and GM-CSF is a growth factor for granulocytes and monocytes. IL-4 is a stimulating factor for both B and T cells and IL-5 is a growth factor for B cells and eosinophils. IL-6 affects the differentiation of B cells into antibody-producing plasma cells and IL-7 acts as a pre-B cell and thymocyte growth factor. Interferon-α affects viral replication and interferon-γ both activates T cells and macrophages and up-regulates the surface expression of class II MHC molecules. Most cytokines produced by T helper cells also affect the growth of hemopoietic cells in the bone marrow. Many cytokine genes have now been cloned and sequenced. The production of recombinant cytokines has opened exciting new avenues both for immunology and for making monoclonal antibodies.

1.3 Self-tolerance and the concept of autoimmunity

Self-tolerance and the ability to discriminate between self and non-self antigens are central to the immune response. If this breaks down the body will react immunologically against itself – that is, autoimmunity will develop. In 1899 Paul Ehrlich considered that autoimmunity was an abnormality the body must avoid and coined the term "horror autotoxicus".

1.3.1 The immunological basis for self–non-self recognition

Immunological tolerance (i.e. the failure to respond to self-antigens) develops *in utero* when immature lymphocytes are exposed to self-antigens. The thymus plays a critical role in educating T lymphocytes to discriminate between self and non-self. Stem cells migrate from sites of general hemopoiesis to the thymus. There they are transformed, after having received a suitable signal, from blastoid cells into a large number of small lymphocytes. An early event in the development of these cells is the rearrangement of TCR genes. TCR γ and δ genes are rearranged first, followed by α and β genes. V, D and J region genes are rearranged into unique combinations and coupled with C region genes. Inevitably some TCR gene rearrangements will recognize self molecules. These need to be eliminated or inactivated.

T lymphocytes undergo intensive selection within the thymus before they are released into the peripheral circulation. Ninety-nine per cent of T cells never leave the thymus. Developing T cells can be deleted from the repertoire by negative selection or amplified by positive selection. Lymphocytes in the thymus go from low to high CD3 surface expression; from being both CD4- and CD8-positive (double positive) to being single positive; and have increasing levels of CD2 surface molecules during the course of development. Negative and positive selection both occur at the double positive stage (*Figure 1.5*).

Negative selection occurs following interaction of the TCR with self-antigen and MHC molecules. Super-antigens such as *Staphylococcus* enterotoxin B can also affect the final T cell repertoire by negative selection. Super-antigens are not presented as processed peptide but can cross-link MHC to TCR Vβ elements. Lymphocyte death in negative selection is thought to occur as a programmed 'self suicide' called apoptosis.

T lymphocytes are positively selected on the basis of having TCRs which can recognize self-MHC. The T cells selected interact with MHC molecules on epithelial cells in the thymus, in the absence of any foreign peptide. Whether a T cell ends up in the CD4- or CD8-positive population depends on whether it interacts with class I or class II MHC molecules. Thus one role of the thymus is to split T cells into the two major functional subclasses: helper and suppressor/cytotoxic.

How the thymus manages to turn MHC recognition and antigen presentation from providing negative selection at one stage to positive selection at another is unclear. It is thought that the type of antigen presenting cell in the thymus and its affinity for antigen may be critical in determining the selection process involved and dictate whether T cells are given the 'kiss of death' or the 'kiss of life'. Development of the T cell repertoire is largely dependent on which cells the thymus leaves untouched. By subjecting T cells to such a stringent process the immune system selects cells which are 'obsessed' with self-MHC but are unable to recognize self-MHC-presenting self-

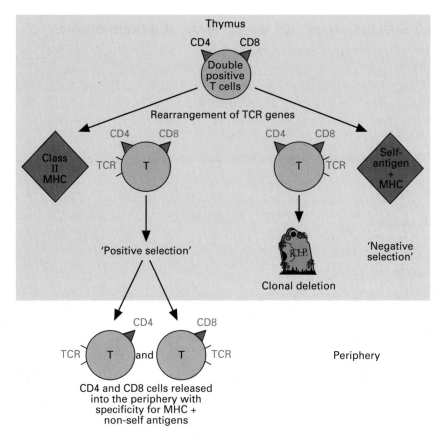

Figure 1.5: *Positive and negative selection of T cells.*

peptide (auto-antigen) encountered at later stages of ontogeny. This also explains why administration of 'foreign' antigen at an early stage in ontogeny can result in clonal deletion and subsequent unresponsiveness to the antigen.

   B cells cannot usually discriminate self from non-self. Like the TCR, immunoglobulin genes are the result of rearrangements of V, D, J and C segment genes. Superimposed on this rearrangement is a high degree of somatic mutation, resulting in a vast repertoire of antibody–antigen combining sites. Thus antibodies will inevitably be produced which are capable of recognizing self-antigens. However, as described in Section 1.2.1, most antibody production will only occur if the T helper cell is also activated by self-antigen. It is thought that B cells can themselves be made tolerant by exposure to non-physiological concentrations of antigens in the absence of T cells.

1.3.2 Peripheral tolerance

Occasionally T cells reactive against a particular self-antigen may escape detection in the thymus. In this situation peripheral tolerance is a second line of protection against self-recognition. Certain *in-vitro* manipulations will encourage unresponsive T cells to respond to self-antigen. Peripheral tolerance is thought to be mediated largely by CD8-positive T cells. Suppressor T cells can actively 'turn off' other T lymphocytes in an antigen-specific manner. Such cells are part of a complex circuit of regulatory cells with an overall function of negative feedback on the immune response. CD8 cytotoxic cells may either kill the stimulating cells or consume interleukins necessary for a response. Alternatively, CD8-positive cells may kill specific CD4 cells in a type of T cell idiotype network through recognition of TCRs.

1.3.3 Ageing and the decline in self-tolerance

Epidemiological evidence indicates an increased prevalence of autoimmune diseases, cancer and infections in old age. These phenomena are attributed to a decline in immune surveillance so that the immune system begins to make mistakes – it fails to eliminate harmful organisms and malignant cells, and is more likely to react against self-antigens.

A number of changes in immune function are seen in the ageing process. The thymus involutes. Fewer pre-T cells enter the thymus and yet it comprises a greater proportion of immature T cells. The number of circulating helper T cells falls and there is impaired proliferative capacity of T cells. Similarly, older individuals produce lower levels of antibodies following immunization. Yet serum IgG and IgA levels tend to rise, while IgM and IgE fall. There is an increased appearance of auto-antibodies – up to 16% of individuals over the age of 70 have antinuclear antibodies.

1.4 Theories concerning the development of autoimmunity

Autoimmunity develops following a loss of self-tolerance. A range of explanations for the phenomenon have been put forward. Any acceptable hypothesis must be compatible with what is already known about the genetic (Chapter 2) and environmental (Chapter 3) factors and with the observation that autoimmunity is more prevalent in females and increases with advancing age. Many of the theories mentioned here are dealt with in more detail later.

1.4.1 Presentation of sequestered self-antigens

The self-antigens of a few body constituents are hidden from the lymphoreticular system. As a result immunological tolerance is not established and potentially self-reactive T cells are not eliminated. This situation appears to apply to the lens of the eye, to sperm and to heart tissue. When these tissues are damaged or, in the case of the lens, vascularized, an autoimmune response can ensue. Autoimmune orchitis following mumps infection and sympathetic ophthalmitis are examples of such responses. This explanation cannot be given as a general basis for developing autoimmunity as most organ-specific antigens are exposed to the immune system.

1.4.2 Cross-reactivity

Cross-reactivity may exist between a self-antigen and exogenous antigens, perhaps expressed by an infecting micro-organism (Section 3.2.1). If this cross-reactive or shared epitope is presented to the immune system in the context of a different carrier, helper T cells will give a suitable signal to any B cells with antibody receptors recognizing the epitope.

1.4.3 Modification of auto-antigens – altered self

Auto-antigens can be modified by the action of drugs and chemicals. Alternatively, an endogenous modification of antigen may arise spontaneously due to a defect in a metabolic process. If sufficiently different, the altered antigen could be recognized by TCRs expressed on undeleted T cells, provoking an immune response. The change in the molecule may provide a new carrier sufficient for T helper cells to instruct B cells to proceed with an antibody response to self-antigen. As the immune response is recognizing altered self-antigen these situations cannot be regarded as a classical breakdown in self-tolerance.

1.4.4 Viral infections

Auto-antibodies can sometimes arise following viral infections. It is thought that the addition of a new viral antigen on the cell surface and the T cell response this can induce may, in some circumstances, be sufficient to induce a response to a pre-existing cell component. The mechanism for this 'innocent bystander' effect is not understood.

1.4.5 Inappropriate or ectopic expression of HLA class II antigens

In normal circumstances class II MHC antigens have a restricted tissue distribution. However, in autoimmune diseases the tissue to which the response is mounted may express class II antigens inappropriately. Such expression may be a critical step in the pathway initiating autoimmunity. One hypothesis suggests that a tissue-specific viral infection induces a localized immune response and the production of γ-interferon (this cytokine induces the expression of class II antigens). A process may therefore be started whereby tissue-specific or differentiation antigens can be presented in the context of class II molecules to an immune response which has never experienced, and thus never eliminated, self-reactive clones to these antigens.

1.4.6 Regulatory defects

Suppressor T cells. T cells may sometimes recognize self-antigen but fail to respond to and co-operate with B cells due to peripheral tolerance exerted by suppressor T cells. A failure in this regulatory mechanism could result in autoimmunity. Evidence from animal models indicates that there may be a progressive loss of T suppressor cell function with age (Section 1.3.3). A second possible explanation for the loss of suppressor T cell activity is the existence of specific contra-suppressor cells.

Idiotype bypass. Viral or environmental antigens may stimulate B cells which express and produce antibodies which have a public epitope (binding site) which is shared with the receptor of other B or T cells which are potentially autoreactive. Such antibodies could provoke and drive an autoimmune response by activating these cells.

Polyclonal B cell activation. For most antigens B cells are under T cell control. However, certain agents can mimic the T cell stimulus and activate B cells to divide polyclonally. They do this either by direct activation of B cells or by stimulating the production of cytokines by T cells and/or macrophages. Such polyclonal stimulation could lead to the activation of B cells secreting auto-antibodies. Bacterial endotoxins such as lipopolysaccharide and a mitogen extract from pokeweed can stimulate B cells non-specifically. The development of autoimmunity by non-specific B cell activation should be limited by the presence of the inducing agent and cease once the stimulus is withdrawn. The chronic presence of B cell activators such as Epstein–Barr virus (Section 3.2.3) (or other viruses) may be more relevant to the development of autoimmunity. B lymphocytes taken from rheumatoid arthritis (RA), systemic lupus erythematosus (SLE) and Sjögren's Syndrome (SS) patients will often transform spontaneously *in vitro* into immortalized polyclonal B cell lines. This suggests that some form of polyclonal activation process is also operating *in vivo*. Auto-antibodies and rheumatoid factors are often secreted by such immortalized polyclonal B cell lines.

1.5 The clinical spectrum of autoimmunity

There is a remarkable range of autoimmune diseases. Almost every system of the body may be involved in an autoimmune process. These diseases are described in detail in Chapters 5 and 6. The spectrum of autoimmune disease spans conditions with involvement of a single organ (e.g. Hashimoto's thyroiditis) through to those with involvement of all systems in the body (e.g. SLE) (*Figure 1.6*). The distribution of the auto-antigen largely determines the manifestations of the disease.

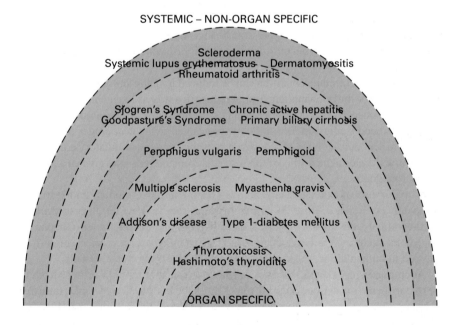

Figure 1.6: *The spectrum of autoimmune disease.*

1.6 Clustering of autoimmune diseases

In the non-organ-specific autoimmune diseases there is often an overlap of auto-antibody profiles and clinical features in the same individual. Thus a patient may present with some features of SLE and some features of scleroderma and is said to have an 'overlap syndrome'. It is also possible for the same individual to have two quite different autoimmune diseases (e.g. thyroid disease and rheumatoid arthritis) simultaneously. This happens far more frequently than one would expect by chance. Similarly there may be clustering of autoimmune diseases within the same family. This phenomenon can be explained in part by the underlying genetic basis of these diseases (Chapter 2) but this does not account for one sister in a sibship developing pernicious anemia while another develops Hashimoto's thyroiditis.

1.7 Animal models of autoimmunity

Research into autoimmunity has been furthered greatly by the use of disease models in animals. Various species have been used but the majority of models relate to inbred strains of mice and rats. A representative selection is summarized in *Table 1.1*. Animal models can be informative about a variety of aspects of disease (*Table 1.2*). Ideally such models should be disease-specific, exhibit clinical and immunological features representative of the analogous human condition and be reproducible both in the way they are induced and in the clinical features manifested. Disease models may occur spontaneously or be induced by experimental procedures.

Spontaneous models provide an excellent basis for studying the genetics of disease susceptibility. Environmental triggers can be investigated in strains of animals which are genetically susceptible but only develop the disease when experimentally manipulated in some way.

A specific autoimmune condition can be induced in many animals by the artificial administration of the relevant (auto)antigen in such a way as to encourage a vigorous immune response. This usually necessitates the use of a strong adjuvant such as complete Freund's adjuvant. It is not clear how an adjuvant encourages the immune response to see 'auto-antigen' as foreign but strong immunostimulatory components such as mycobacterial heat shock proteins and super-antigens may give an additional necessary signal.

A major use of animal disease models is in the development and testing of therapeutic compounds. In addition such models provide an opportunity to work out the theoretical and practical aspects of new immunotherapies (see Chapter 7). Procedures such as T cell vaccination and induction of oral tolerance can only be assessed in human clinical trials after exhaustive testing in animal models.

An important area of potential future research into autoimmunity comes from the use of transgenic mice. Such mice are obtained by the transfection of genes, human or otherwise (e.g. potential disease susceptibility genes, TCR genes, MHC genes, immunoglobulin genes) into inbred mouse strain embryos, with the result that full-grown animals express a human gene in adult mouse tissues. Once genetically engineered, the mice can be bred as a true line. In this way the relevance and effects of single genes can be assessed.

Transgenic mice have been used in cancer studies, but they also have an application in autoimmunity. Much information about positive and negative selection of T cells in

Table 1.1: *Animal models of autoimmunity*

Disease model	Animal	Inducing agent	Clinical features
Autoimmune thyroiditis	OS chicken Buffalo rat CBA mouse	Spontaneous Spontaneous Experimentally induced in CFA[a] with thyroglobulin	Thyroiditis with lymphoid infiltration and follicular destruction
Experimental myasthenia gravis	Susceptible mouse and rat strains	Experimentally induced by injection with acetyl choline receptor (autologous or from electric fish)	Impaired nerve conductivity, MG-like condition
Experimental autoimmune encephalomyelitis (multiple sclerosis)	Susceptible mouse and rat strains	Injection with myelin basic protein	MS-like condition
Type I diabetes mellitus	NOD (non-obese diabetic) mouse, BB rat	Spontaneous	Insulin-dependent diabetes secondary to islet β cell destruction following infiltration by lymphoid cells
Autoimmune hemolytic anemia	NZB mouse	Spontaneous	Hemolytic anemia Coombs-positive antibodies Nephropathy
Systemic lupus erythematosus	MLR/1 mouse NZW/NZB mouse	Spontaneous in homozygotes Spontaneous	Raised IgG, IgM circulating immune complexes, auto-antibodies, splenomegaly, glomerulonephritis
Systemic sclerosis (scleroderma)	Tight skin mouse	Spontaneous in heterozygotes (homozygotes die *in utero*)	Excessive deposition of type I collagen in skin and internal organs
Arthritis	Rats–various strains	Adjuvant induced – CFA[a] (mycobacterial extracts in oil emulsion)	Polyarthritis
		Pristane induced (mineral oil)	Polyarthritis
	Rats (Lewis, Sprague-Dawley)	Type II collagen induced (human, bovine, chick, mouse collagen)	Duration 1–2 months, abrupt onset in hind and fore paws
	Rats (various strains)	Streptococcal cell wall fragments	Erosive synovitis
	Goats	Spontaneous virally induced caprine arthritis encephalitis virus (retrovirus)	Progressive arthritis and leukoencephalomyelitis

[a]CFA – complete Freund's adjuvant.

Table 1.2: *Information gained from disease models in animals*

Drug testing
Genetic susceptibility
Pathology and course of disease
Models for immunotherapy (T cell vaccination, oral tolerance, etc.)
Genetic – environmental interaction
Identification and manipulation of disease genes
Immune response to epitopes within auto-antigens

the thymus and generation of the T cell repertoire has come from studies using these animals. HLA transgenic mice offer the possibility of establishing mouse models of HLA linked diseases, for example, the association between HLA-B27 and ankylosing spondylitis is being studied in this way. HLA-B27 transgenic mice are more susceptible to infection with *Yersinia enterocolitica* than untransfected animals and a proportion develop paralysis of the hind legs. NOD mice (which develop Type I-DM spontaneously) are also being transfected with different H-2 MHC genes to assess the protection afforded by such genes.

1.8 Conclusion

This chapter has described the role and structure of the immune system and has introduced the concept of autoimmunity. The basis for autoimmunity lies in the failure of self-recognition and a breakdown of self-tolerance. This may occur for a variety of reasons, although the main cause is assumed to lie at the level of immune regulation. It is important to stress that no satisfactory explanation for autoimmunity exists as yet. Nevertheless, recent advances in molecular biology, when applied to autoimmunity, are providing important insights into these conditions. Research into autoimmunity has also been furthered greatly by the use of disease models in animals. The remainder of this book concerns the genetic, immunological and clinical diversity of the phenomenon of autoimmunity.

Further reading

Arnold, B., Goodnow, C., Hengartner, H. and Hammerling, G. (1990) The coming of transgenic mice: tolerance and immune reactivity. *Immunol. Today,* **11**, 69.

Blackwell, T.K. and Alt, F. (1988) Immunoglobulin genes. in *Molecular Immunology.* Frontiers in Molecular Biology Series (Hames, B.D. and Glover, D.M., eds). IRL Press, Oxford, p.1.

Davis, M.M. (1988) T cell antigen receptor genes. in *Molecular Immunology.* Frontiers in Molecular Biology Series (Hames, B.D. and Glover, D.M., eds). IRL Press, Oxford, p. 61.

Festing, M.F.H. (1979) *Inbred Strains in Biomedical Research.* Macmillan, London.

Greenwald, R.A. and Diamond, H.S. (1988) *CRC Handbook of Animal Models for the Rheumatic Disease*, Vol. 1. CRC Press, Florida.

Hopkins, S.J. (1990) Cytokines and their significance in rheumatic disease. in *Anti-rheumatic Drugs* (M. C. L. Orme, ed.). Pergamon, New York, p. 49.

Klein, J.(1982) *Immunology. The Science of Self–Nonself Discrimination.* John Wiley, New York.

O'Garra, A. (1989) Interleukins and the immune system. *Lancet*, **1**, 943.

Pereira, P., Bandeira, A., Continho, A., Marcos, M.A., Toribio, M. and Martinez, C. (1989) V-region connectivity in T cell repertoires. *Ann. Rev. Immunol.*, **7**, 209.

Raulet, D.H. (1989) The structure, function and molecular genetics of the γ/δ T cell receptor. *Ann. Rev. Immunol.*, **7**, 175.

Roitt, I., Brostoff, J. and Male, D. (1985) *Immunology*. Churchill Livingstone, Edinburgh.

Schwartz, R.H. (1989) Acquisition of immunologic self-tolerance. *Cell*, **57**, 1073.

Stites, D.P., Stobo, J.D., Fudenberg, H.H. and Wells, J.V. (1990) *Basic and Clinical Immunology*. Appleton and Lange, Norwalk, Connecticut.

Williamson, A.R. and Turner, M.W. (1978) *Essential Immunogenetics*. Blackwell Scientific Publications, Oxford.

Wraith, D.C., McDevitt, H.O., Steinman, L. and Acha-Orbea, H. (1989) T cell recognition as the target for immune intervention in autoimmune disease. *Cell*, **57**, 709.

2
THE GENETIC BASIS OF AUTOIMMUNE DISEASE

2.1 Introduction

A genetic component is suspected in the etiology of many autoimmune diseases because of their tendency to cluster in families. Indeed genetic encoded susceptibility may be a feature of all autoimmunity. However, the problems in analyzing this genetic basis are immense and complex. As yet no autoimmune disease has been shown to be due to a single gene defect and it is likely that most, if not all, such diseases have a polygenic basis. As the study of genetics in autoimmune disease is difficult, mainstream genetic research has largely been directed to diseases associated with classical single gene defects and known modes of transmission, such as Duchenne muscular dystrophy and cystic fibrosis. Recent advances in molecular biology have, however, provided new approaches which can be applied to autoimmune diseases enabling clinicians, immunogeneticists and molecular biologists to start making inroads into understanding disease susceptibility.

Identification of disease susceptibility genes would have two applications. First the information might be used to identify individuals at risk of a particular disease; or to identify sub-sets of patients likely to respond well to a particular therapy or to follow a certain prognostic course. Secondly, the genes and their products could be characterized to see how they relate to the disease pathology. Depending on its role, the gene product it might either be supplemented or antagonized as treatment of the disease.

2.2 How do we know there is a genetic basis for autoimmunity?

The evidence for a role for genetic factors in autoimmune diseases has come from various types of study, as described below.

2.2.1 Family studies

Many autoimmune diseases appear to cluster in families. This familial tendency is seen clearly in thyroid disease, Type I-diabetes mellitus (TI-DM) and rheumatoid arthritis (RA), where close relatives of patients have a higher chance of developing the disease than age-matched controls. Clustering of different autoimmune diseases may also be seen in the same family (*Figure 2.1*). This is frequently observed between RA

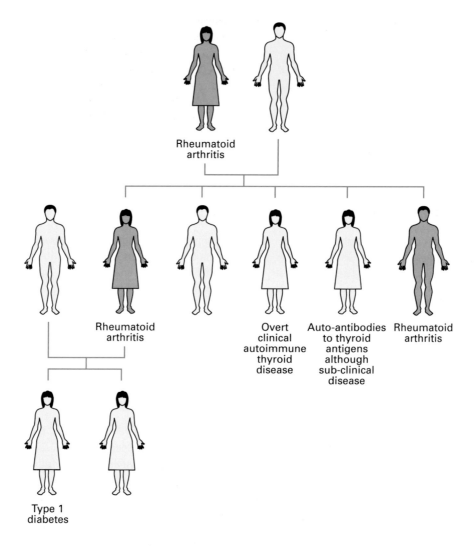

Figure 2.1: *Pedigree of a family with autoimmune disease.*

and thyroid disease, and between RA and TI-DM. This suggests that a 'common genetic denominator' may exist in such families. Family studies are also important in identifying and tracking putative disease susceptibility genes. The most useful families are those with extended pedigrees containing multiple affected cases.

2.2.2 Twin studies

Twin studies are the classical way of identifying genetic susceptibility and estimating the relative contributions of genetic and environmental factors in the etiology of a disease. A standard approach is to examine the frequency of both twins being affected (disease concordance) in identical (monozygotic – MZ) and non-identical (dizygotic – DZ) twins. Monozygotic twins inherit identical germline DNA and therefore share any disease susceptibility genes. A disease concordance rate that is higher in MZ twins than in DZ twins indicates that there is a significant genetic component. Theoretically if there is a genetic basis for a disease, the disease concordance in identical twins should be 100%. However, this is never the case, as disease susceptibility genes may not be fully penetrant (Section 2.3.1) and need an environmental trigger to exhibit the disease phenotype. Twin studies can, therefore, also be used to estimate the environmental component and penetrance of genes. For example, in RA approximately 30% concordance is observed in MZ twins compared to 11% in DZ pairs. Thus while this disease clearly has a genetic basis there is also a major environmental component. Twin studies have not been performed on all autoimmune conditions. A selection are detailed in *Table 2.1*.

Table 2.1: Concordance of autoimmune diseases in MZ and DZ twins

	MZ	DZ
Rheumatoid arthritis	32%	11%
Systemic lupus erythematosus	57%	?
Multiple sclerosis	25%	2%
Type I diabetes mellitus	50%	5%
Hyperthyroidism	47%	3%
Myasthenia gravis		Case reports of
Pernicious anemia		co-affection in
Idiopathic Addison's disease		MZ pairs

2.2.3 Population studies

Evidence for a genetic basis of autoimmunity has also come from demonstrating an association between specific genes and disease at the population level. The most clear associations have been demonstrated with genes inside the MHC (Section 2.5). These associations range from weak to very strong and provide clear evidence for the existence of a genetic component to these diseases. Other associations have been observed with genes encoding immunoglobulin heavy chains (Gm allotypes) and components of the T cell receptor.

2.3 What are the problems associated with genetic analysis of autoimmune disease?

2.3.1 Genetic problems

Polygenic diseases. All autoimmune diseases are probably polygenic. This means that the overall inheritance of the disease will not follow Mendelian laws and, as the number of genes and how they interact together is unknown, it is difficult to study one gene in isolation from the others.

Incomplete penetrance. The genetic constitution of an individual is termed the genotype. The characteristics manifested by the individual make up the phenotype. When a given genotype is always expressed in such a way as to give a certain phenotype, the gene is said to be completely penetrant. When the disease phenotype is only expressed in a proportion of the individuals carrying the gene, it is said to have reduced or incomplete penetrance. For such genes the way the environment acts is very important in determining how they are expressed. Estimating the penetrance of genes can be extremely difficult and when many genes are involved the proportion of subjects expressing the disease phenotype may represent an overall penetrance of a number of genes each with its own penetrance.

Mode of transmission. For polygenic diseases it is impossible to say that a disease is inherited in a dominant or recessive manner. These terms can only be applied to individual genes. Polygenic disease can only be interpreted in the light of the inheritance pattern of all genetic factors and their penetrance. For example, if two fully penetrant genes A and B are both needed to develop the disease, the first in a recessive manner, the second dominant, it might be thought that the genotype *AaBb* would be enough for the disease to develop. However, the genotype *AaBb* will not result in disease because although *B* is dominantly inherited the individual has only inherited one A gene and not the two needed to express the disease recessively.

2.3.2 Epidemiological problems

Age at disease onset and status miss-assignment. Autoimmunity increases in prevalence with age. For some diseases this creates a problem for case ascertainment in family studies. A good contrast is seen between TI-DM and RA. In TI-DM families one can be relatively certain that, by the age of 35 years, everyone likely to develop TI-DM will have done so. Family members above this age can therefore confidently be differentiated into affected and non-affected individuals. In contrast, the mean age of onset of RA is around 45 and the disease may develop even at the age of 80 or 90. The assignment of members into affected and non-affected will, therefore, apply to one point in time and there may be 'unaffected' family members carrying the gene(s), who will develop the disease in later life. Miss-assignment introduces a large source of error in subsequent genetic analysis. Similarly it may be difficult confidently to assign disease status due to the presence of more than one condition in the patient or to there being cases with mild disease not satisfying diagnostic criteria.

Selection of pedigrees. The ideal families for genetic analysis are both extended and contain many affected members. The frequency of such families is largely dependent on how common the disease is in the population (i.e. the disease prevalence). Such families can be difficult to find for the rarer autoimmune conditions and a concerted effort is often required. A related problem has been the increasing tendency towards smaller sibships in many countries. The age at disease onset also limits how extensive pedigrees will be for some diseases. For example with RA, which has a relatively late mean age at onset, the parents of most patients will no longer be alive.

2.4 Analysis of disease susceptibility

Given a possible marker or candidate disease susceptibility gene it is important to ascertain whether linkage exists between the gene and the condition (i.e. whether both are encoded by the same area of the chromosome). Linkage can be detected up to approximately 10^7 base pairs either side of the disease susceptibility gene. Various methods of analysis can be used, the better known methods being LOD score analysis and affected sibling pair ratio analysis.

2.4.1 LOD score analysis

This analysis examines all of the pedigree data including affected and non-affected individuals. If the candidate gene and the disease gene are not linked there is a 50% chance of the two segregating together in the same individual. The logarithm of the odds (LOD) of finding the two together on the same chromosome is therefore calculated. A LOD score greater than 3 is taken to indicate significant linkage (i.e. odds of 1 in 1000). For this analysis the penetrance of the disease gene has to be estimated and LOD scores can be calculated for a range of recombination distances between the two genes. The mode of transmission is also an important variable and linkage is examined for both dominant and recessive models. LOD score analysis is complicated and best carried out using a computer program. The disadvantages of LOD score analysis are: first, that gene penetrance and recombination distance have to be estimated; and secondly, that the method is sensitive to misclassification of disease status in family members.

2.4.2 Affected sibling pair ratio analysis

This method is simpler to understand and perform than LOD score analysis. It is based on the inheritance of chromosomal haplotypes by affected sibling pairs (a haplotype is the information encoded by one of a pair of chromosomes; thus there are two distinct haplotypes for each pair). Siblings may have two, one or zero haplotypes in common, at frequencies of 25%, 50% and 25% respectively (*Figure 2.2*). This distribution can therefore be examined for a candidate gene and a disease in sibling pairs who are both affected. Any distortion of the distribution towards greater haplotype sharing indicates linkage between the gene and the condition. To perform such an analysis a large number of affected sibling pairs is needed. The advantage of this method is that gene penetrance can be ignored as only affected cases are considered. A disadvantage is that most of the pedigree data are not utilized.

2.5 The HLA system

A major piece of the 'autoimmune jigsaw' became apparent when it was realized that MHC encoded products were implicated in the susceptibility to many diseases. The MHC comprises a set of tightly linked genes on the short arm of chromosome 6. It is more often referred to as the HLA system (human leucocyte antigens). A simplified diagrammatic representation of the chromosomal organization of the HLA system is given in *Figure 2.3*. A more detailed plan of this region has been reported by Trowsdale *et al.* (see Further reading).

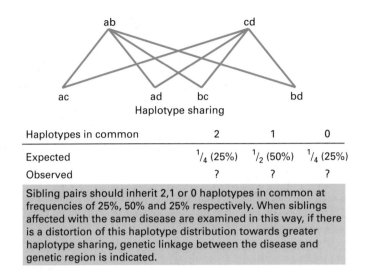

Haplotypes in common	2	1	0
Expected	$^1/_4$ (25%)	$^1/_2$ (50%)	$^1/_4$ (25%)
Observed	?	?	?

Sibling pairs should inherit 2,1 or 0 haplotypes in common at frequencies of 25%, 50% and 25% respectively. When siblings affected with the same disease are examined in this way, if there is a distortion of this haplotype distribution towards greater haplotype sharing, genetic linkage between the disease and genetic region is indicated.

Figure 2.2: *Affected sibling pair method.*

2.5.1 HLA antigens – classification

HLA genes have been divided into three classes. The class I region may contain as many as 17 gene loci although only three, HLA-A, -B and -C have been well-characterized. These molecules consist of two non-covalently associated polypeptide chains, one being the polymorphic transmembrane glycosylated heavy chain and the

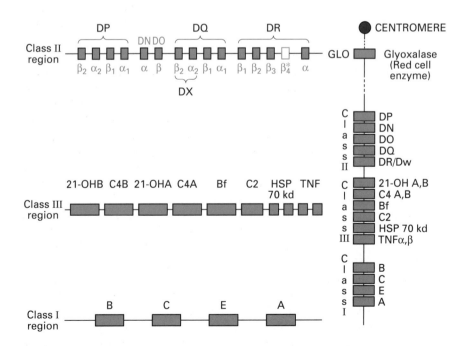

Figure 2.3: *The HLA system – chromosome 6.*

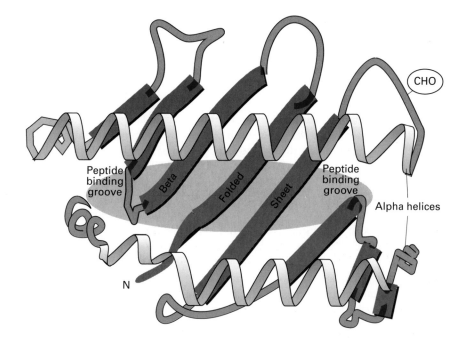

Figure 2.4: *Representation of MHC molecule.*

other a non-polymorphic, non-transmembrane β_2-microglobulin light chain (encoded on chromosome 15). Class I antigens are expressed on the surface of virtually all nucleated cells. The class I molecule (HLA-A2) has been crystallized and the three-dimensional structure deduced (*Figure 2.4*).

Genes in the MHC complex are co-dominantly expressed and typified by their extreme polymorphism, with many different alleles being possible for each locus. Alleles of different loci are found in the population at certain frequencies. For example, the allele HLA-A1 is relatively common and has a gene frequency of 0.2 (20%) in Caucasians. Similarly the allele HLA-B8 is found at a frequency of 0.15. In addition most genes strongly exhibit the phenomenon of linkage disequilibrium. The expected frequency of finding the two antigens HLA-A1 and B8 together can be calculated as the product of their individual frequencies ($0.2 \times 0.15 = 0.03$). However, in many cases the observed frequency of finding alleles from different loci together is much higher than expected. These alleles are then said to be in linkage disequilibrium.

HLA class II region molecules are also heterodimers consisting of non-covalently associated transmembrane, glycosylated α and β chains. The external domains of these chains are the main sites for polymorphic determinants. Within the class II region are the DR, DQ and DP sub-regions. For DR there are up to five β genes (depending on the haplotype) and one non-polymorphic α gene. The DRβ gene specifies the poly-morphic determinants of the original DR antigenic series (DR1 – DRw16). Other DRβ genes encode the DRw52 and DRw53 specificities. HLA-DR antigens contain epitopes which can stimulate 'foreign' T cells to divide in mixed lymphocyte culture. This is referred to as an alloreactive response. T cells can recognize even subtle differences within the DRβ_1 specificities. For example, T cell responses can divide DR4 into at least five different sub-types; Dw4, Dw10, Dw13, Dw14 and Dw15.

Historically, these specificities have been referred to as HLA-Dw types and could only be detected by cellular methods. More recently the molecular bases for these Dw types have been identified and their amino acid sequences deduced. The differences tend to be found in the first domain of $DR\beta_1$ and they can now be detected more easily using allele-specific oligonucleotide probes.

The HLA-DQ subregion includes two α and two β chain genes. Only one α/β pair encodes the DQ serological specificities. The other pair, although polymorphic at the DNA level, are 'pseudo-genes'. DQ α and β genes are both polymorphic. HLA-DP determinants were originally discovered through primed lymphocyte typing using T cells activated in HLA-DR/Dw identical combinations. The DNA sequences are now known for many DR, DQ and DP polymorphisms and these are defined more accurately by allele-specific oligonucleotide typing than by serology. The class II molecular structure has not yet been confirmed by crystallographic studies. However, it is thought not to differ significantly from the class I structure. The cell surface molecule is considered to comprise a flat β-sheet on which rest two α-helices. The groove between these two helices contains foreign or self peptide.

Class II antigens have a more restricted tissue distribution, being absent on T lymphocytes and many tissues of the body. They are expressed strongly on B lymphocytes and on antigen presenting cells such as macrophages and dendritic cells. The expression of class II molecules can be up-regulated by a number of cytokines including interferon and tumor necrosis factor. Thus cells not normally expressing class II molecules can be induced to do so by their micro-environment. T lymphocytes also express class II antigens when they are activated.

The class III region proteins are not cell surface antigens but comprise three

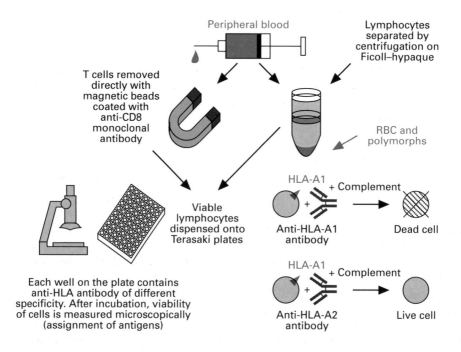

Figure 2.5: Class I HLA typing.

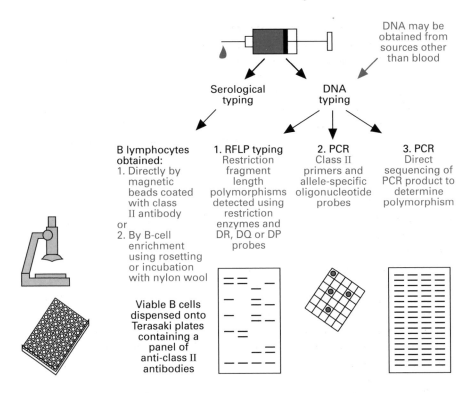

Figure 2.6: *Class II HLA typing.*

complement components, controlled by four closely linked polymorphic genes: C2, BF, C4A and C4B. In addition two genes, 21-OHA and 21-OHB, which regulate the levels of cortisol, are encoded in this region, as well as genes encoding the 70 kd heat shock protein and tumor necrosis factor (TNFα, TNFβ).

2.5.2 Identification of HLA antigens

Class I HLA antigens are routinely identified with serological typing methods. Viable lymphocytes can be obtained from peripheral blood samples by a variety of methods (*Figure 2.5*). Lymphocytes are dispensed into Terasaki typing plates where each individual well contains an antibody of known HLA specificity. After the addition of fresh rabbit serum (as a source of complement), HLA antigens can be assigned depending on which antibodies have reacted with the cells. Cell death is assessed microscopically.

Class II typing can be performed using either serological or DNA typing methods (*Figure 2.6*). Serological methods require purified samples of B lymphocytes (class II positive cells). B cells can be obtained from peripheral blood by incubation with nylon wool, by magnetic bead separation or by T cell depletion through rosetting with sheep red blood cells. Methods for serological class II typing are similar to those described for class I, using Terasaki plates which contain a panel of different anti-class II antibodies, potentially capable of recognizing all class II polymorphisms.

Typing methods using DNA have recently been introduced. A popular method has been restriction enzyme digestion of genomic DNA followed by Southern blotting and probing with DRβ, DQβ and DPβ probes. Each class II antigen tends to have its own characteristic 'signature' or restriction fragment length polymorphism (RFLP) which can be assigned when compared with reference patterns of known HLA type. Following the introduction of the polymerase chain reaction (PCR) (*Figure 2.7*), RFLP typing is being superseded by allele-specific oligonucleotide (ASO) typing (*Figure 2.8*). All of the known class II antigens have now been DNA sequenced. This information provides the basis for designing sequence specific oligonucleotide probes. When the class II genes have been amplified by PCR, the DNA can be blotted onto membrane and incubated with labeled ASO probes. Under stringent washing conditions, hybridization of a probe indicates the presence of the corresponding gene.

The technology used in molecular biology is now advancing so fast that routine

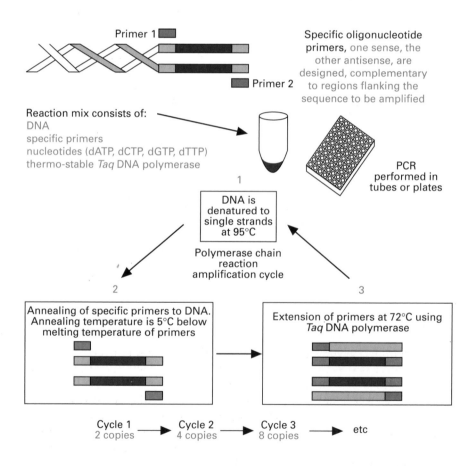

Figure 2.7: The polymerase chain reaction.

HLA typing by the rapid DNA sequencing of PCR amplified HLA genes is becoming a reality.

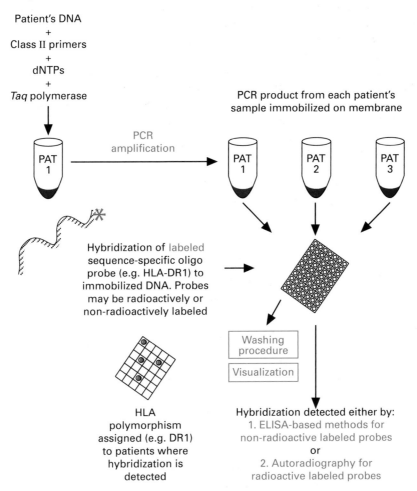

Figure 2.8: *HLA allele-specific oligonucleotide typing.*

2.5.3 The role of HLA

As the name implies, many products of the MHC act as transplantation antigens and as targets for allorecognition in graft rejection. However, this is an artificial situation and undoubtedly this is not their true immunological role.

Class I antigens act primarily as vehicles for presenting foreign peptides to cytotoxic (CD8-positive) T cells. Class II antigens are cell surface molecules which can present foreign peptides to receptors on T cells capable of undergoing clonal expansion and of producing cytokines. T cells activated in these ways provide efficient defense mechanisms, especially against viral infections.

Endogenous peptide (that is, peptide from within the cell) is held in the groove formed by the α-helices of class I HLA antigens. The peptide–class I complexes can then be recognized by CD8-positive cells bearing T cell receptors with the relevant specificity. If this presentation occurs at an early pre-cytotoxic stage the T cell is induced to express the interleukin-2 (IL-2) receptor on its surface. The presence of exogenous IL-2 (from CD4-positive T cells) will induce these cells to undergo clonal expansion. The resulting CD8-positive T cells will be able to destroy any cells with class I MHC antigens presenting the specific peptide antigen. In the case of a virally infected cell, viral antigen will be occupying the class I groove and cytotoxic T cells will 'home' in to destroy the cells and limit the infection. Cytotoxic T cells are only capable of recognizing foreign peptide in the context of their own class I antigens – thus the target and effector cells have to share class I antigens. This is referred to as class I HLA restricted killing.

It is thought that the groove in the class I antigen is never empty and that in normal circumstances it will contain self-peptide. Cytotoxic T cells are not generated to these complexes due to the elimination of self-reacting T cell clones within the thymus early in development. Only when T cell receptors recognize foreign peptide and self class I antigen together, will a cytotoxic reaction occur. As all nucleated cells of the body can act as hosts for virus replication, it becomes apparent why the tissue distribution of class I antigen is almost universal. By employing this system for directing cytotoxic responses, there is a risk of a virus evolving which shares or mimics class I structure. This could enable the virus to escape detection and prove fatal. This may explain why multiple MHC loci and extensive polymorphism have evolved.

The class II molecules also contain foreign or self peptide in the groove between the α-helices. This peptide is not endogenous but exogenous in nature. Peptide can bind directly to class II (probably by displacing the peptide already there), although more often it is taken into the antigen presenting cell and processed by enzymatic degradation before combining with class II antigen and being expressed on the surface. This degradation is thought to be non-lysosomal and mainly by aspartic protease such as cathepsin E. Any class II bearing cell should be capable of presenting foreign peptide to T cells. However, some cells are more efficient than others. Such cells have high levels of cell surface class II expression, a large cell surface area, will efficiently degrade antigen and are effective at pinocytosing or phagocytosing exogenous material. Macrophages and dendritic cells have such qualities and are good antigen presenters.

The peptide–class II complex is recognized by T cells bearing receptors with the relevant specificity. Thus the recognition of foreign antigen specificity is predominantly due to the T cell receptor and not the class II molecule. On recognition of antigen presented in this way, CD4-positive T cells undergo clonal expansion resulting in committed cells which will produce cytokines (especially IL-2).

2.5.4 HLA and disease association

Early studies in the mouse indicated that susceptibility and resistance to a variety of virally induced tumors are encoded by genes within the H-2 complex (H-2 is the MHC of the mouse). This provoked a search for similar associations in man. Initial studies indicated at best only weak associations. However, following the discovery of the strong association between HLA-B27 and ankylosing spondylitis, many more examples of HLA/disease association have been documented. HLA associated diseases can be categorized in a number of ways. The major groups are: autoimmune diseases, malignancies, diseases with a metabolic component or diseases with unknown etiology. Alternatively these diseases may be divided into those with an obvious immune component and those without. The autoimmune conditions comprise the largest group of diseases associated with HLA polymorphisms. HLA/disease associations can be identified by comparing antigen frequencies between panels of unrelated patients and controls. As the frequencies of HLA antigens differ markedly between populations, it is important that patients and controls should be matched. There is also a need for careful diagnosis given the problems of clinical heterogeneity and overlap of autoimmune conditions.

Most studies have only demonstrated that a particular antigen is statistically more frequent in patients than controls. A relative risk can be calculated by dividing the prevalence of the antigen in patients with the disease by the prevalence in controls (*Table 2.2*). The relative risk gives an estimate of how important HLA is as an overall risk factor. In some conditions HLA antigens are only weakly associated with the disease whereas in others a very strong association exists, for example, narcolepsy, where the antigen HLA-DR2 is found in practically all cases. Very few diseases have been shown to be directly linked to genes in the HLA complex. For linkage analysis either LOD score or affected sibling pair methods have to be used (Section 2.4.1 and 2.4.2). The clearest example of linkage is between congenital adrenal hyperplasia (21-hydroxylase deficiency) and genes within the class III region.

Table 2.2: Calculating the relative risk of having a particular HLA gene

	Disease	No disease
HLA-x	a	b
No HLA-x	c	d
Relative risk=	$\dfrac{a}{a+c}$	$\div$ $\dfrac{b}{b+d}$

Autoimmune diseases are usually associated with class II specificities. However, many conditions are associated with class I, II and III polymorphisms and this is usually due to these alleles being in linkage disequilibrium. For example, in multiple sclerosis, the antigens HLA-A3, B7, Cw7 and DR2 are all disease associated. These specificities are commonly found together as an established haplotype or 'supratype', even in the normal population. Many autoimmune diseases are associated with HLA supratypes and they are listed in *Table 2.3*.

If these 'established haplotypes' or 'supratypes' have been maintained because of some evolutionary advantage they have been given, it seems paradoxical that so many autoimmune conditions should be associated with these haplotypes. One possible explanation is that disease-giving mutations (or deletions) have occurred between loci where there is strong linkage disequilibrium, thus 'freezing' the mutation inside the haplotype.

It may be relevant to consider IgA deficiency within this context. IgA deficiency is a common immunological disorder which is found more frequently in patients with the autoimmune diseases SLE, myasthenia gravis and TI-DM. These conditions may

Table 2.3: HLA supratypes associated with autoimmune disease

HLA supratypes	Autoimmune disease
A1 Cw7 B8 DR3(Dw3)	SLE Sjögren's Syndrome TI-DM
A3 Cw7 B7 DR2(Dw2)	Multiple sclerosis Goodpasture's Syndrome
A2 Cw5 B44 DR4	RA
A2 Cw3 B40 DR4	RA
A2 Cw3 B15 DR4	RA TI-DM
A26 B38 DR4(Dw10)	Pemphigus vulgaris

all share a genetically determined defect encoded within certain HLA-A1-B8-DR3 'supratypes'. The regulation of B cell proliferation, antibody production and IgA, IgG subclass levels has yet to be completely established. However, it is known that various cytokines (non-MHC encoded) and certain MHC encoded products can affect immunoglobulin production. It is therefore possible that antibody regulation and some antibody mediated autoimmune diseases may be due to defects encoded within these HLA 'supratypes'.

Further details of the genetic associations of autoimmune diseases are discussed in Chapters 5 and 6.

2.5.5 The role of HLA in the development of autoimmunity

The role of HLA in the development of autoimmunity has to be considered carefully. Does HLA determine the specificity of the disease process and the trigger which is involved? Or does HLA determine the progression, duration and severity of the disease process? These two possibilities are hard to differentiate, as the development of a disease to the point of the clinical threshold for diagnosis will probably include components for both specificity/initial susceptibility and an additional component for progression and severity. A number of different hypotheses to explain the association of HLA with disease have been put forward, three of which are considered below.

Could HLA antigens act as receptors for a specific virus? This suggestion was one of the earlier explanations for HLA/disease associations. The cell surface HLA molecule could act as a receptor for a specific virus and provide a way for it to infect the cell, thus making individuals carrying a particular gene susceptible. Several instances have been described in the mouse where H-2 molecules can bind specifically to viruses (e.g. Semliki forest virus and adenovirus type II). No specific examples are known in man for HLA being a viral receptor. However, it is clear that cell surface markers in man, such as CD4, can act in this capacity (e.g. as receptor for human immunodeficiency virus – HIV).

This hypothesis would explain the genetic and environmental components in the etiology of many diseases. However, as HLA molecules are not tissue-specific, it does not explain the restricted tissue and auto-antigen specificity of most autoimmune responses. If the virus additionally required a tissue-specific receptor for infection, a restricted response would ensue, causing destruction of the tissue. However, this would then be 'normal' cytotoxicity of virally infected self cells and not an autoimmune response in the classical sense with recognition of auto-antigen. If this hypothesis was modified, so that the virus also shared an epitope with an auto-antigen, both the association of HLA and specific response to auto-antigen could be explained.

Molecular mimicry. It has been suggested that identity or immunological cross-reactivity can exist between HLA molecules and peptide epitopes of a disease-triggering virus or other etiological agent. In this situation, when the peptide is presented to the T cell receptor, the cell could fail to recognize the antigen, possibly resulting in chronic disease. Alternatively, the immune response to the virus could lead to recognition and response to self-MHC antigen. The first possibility does not explain the development of autoimmune responses. In addition the offending organism would carry and express a multitude of other non-cross-reactive epitopes which would serve the purpose of directing a specific immune response. The second explanation is also defective in that a response to self MHC molecules, with a widespread tissue distribution, does not explain recognition of auto-antigen and tissue specificity of most autoimmune disease.

A refinement of this explanation has been put forward by Benjamin and Parham (see Further reading). Using HLA-B27 and ankylosing spondylitis as a model, they suggest that this disease is the result of a cytotoxic T cell response to a peptide only found at the affected tissue site. This peptide can be specifically bound and presented by HLA-B27. Under normal circumstances the self peptide is presented at levels too low for T cell recognition to give either clonal deletion or to mount an immune response. A bacterium or virus may express an epitope which cross-reacts with this peptide. Infection could then lead to high levels of cross-reactive peptide with an affinity for B27 being presented, thus sensitizing T cells and initiating an immune response.

This model could be applied equally well to autoimmune diseases where auto-antigens with preferential MHC binding are normally only expressed at low concentrations and autoreactive clones have never been detected. Pathogens with epitopes in common with auto-antigen could then lead to an autoreactive, antigen-specific response.

One problem with this explanation is the apparent promiscuity of MHC molecules in their binding and presentation of self and foreign peptides.

Immune response genes. Another explanation put forward for the association between HLA and autoimmune diseases is the presence of immune response genes. The MHC genes associated with the disease may act as immune response genes themselves, or may be markers for other immune response genes in linkage disequilibrium.

The ability to respond to an antigen may lie at the level of T cell recognition and so lack of response may be due to a 'hole' in the T cell receptor repertoire. However, class II molecules may be involved and studies in the mouse reveal that the level of immune response to certain well-defined or synthetic antigens can be mapped to the

MHC class II region. A hypo- or hyper-response could depend on both the MHC genotype and on which antigen was being tested. The regulation of immune response may, therefore, also lie at the level of antigen presentation. The possibilities exist that certain class II molecules may have either a high or low affinity for a particular peptide, or may even be incapable of binding to it. Experimental evidence does not favor this as a general explanation for the immune response. In contrast to the final T cell response which is quite specific, most studies point to class II antigens being completely promiscuous in their ability to bind and present processed peptides. The general level of association/disassociation (affinity) between peptide and class II molecules is considered to be much less than for antibody–antigen interactions. This makes biological sense and it is difficult to imagine any micro-organism escaping detection by having antigens that could not be presented. Furthermore, possessing multiple class II genes would help to overcome this possibility.

Although class II antigens appear to be able to present most peptides it is possible that a particular self or non-self antigen may bind to a class II molecule to such an extent as to influence a T cell response to a level capable of provoking an autoimmune response.

Classic experiments in the H-2^{bm12} inbred mouse strain have shown evidence that subtle differences in class II molecules can have a major influence on immune response. The H-2^{bm12} mouse strain differs from the wild-type H-2^b mouse by only three amino acid residues in the third hypervariable region of an Iaβ chain. However, these changes are sufficient to alter greatly the pattern of immune responses seen between the two strains. The H-2^{bm12} mouse is a high responder to sheep insulin but a low responder to beef insulin. The wild-type H-2^b mouse has the opposite pattern of response. Furthermore, the H-2^{bm12} strain is resistant to experimentally induced myasthenia gravis, whereas the wild-type mice are susceptible to this condition. These data may be of great relevance to our understanding of human autoimmune diseases associated with amino acid differences in the third hypervariable region of DRβ$_1$ (e.g. RA).

It is also possible that class II molecules may influence the level of immune response by means other than antigen presentation. A number of situations have been reported where products of the DQ locus are involved in the generation of suppression to specific antigens. It has been suggested that DQ genes are involved more in regulation than in antigen presentation and as such their role in autoimmunity should be studied further.

2.6 Association of autoimmunity with non-MHC encoded genes

Most diseases do not approach a 100% association with HLA antigens. Besides environmental factors this may, in part, be explained by disease heterogeneity or by the presence of, as yet undiscovered, shared HLA epitopes. A more likely explanation is the presence of non-MHC encoded risk factors. A number of associations between autoimmune diseases and genes on chromosome 14 have been reported. These associations are with immunoglobulin heavy chain constant domain genes (Gm allotypes), T cell receptor α chain genes, the gene for the protease inhibitor α$_1$-antitrypsin (PI), and with other polymorphic DNA markers (e.g. D14S1).

2.6.1 Immunoglobulin Gm allotypes

The genes coding for the heavy chains of immunoglobulin are located on chromosome 14. Allotypic variation is found in the constant regions of the heavy chains of IgG_1, IgG_2, IgG_3, IgA_2 and IgE molecules. They are called G1m, G2m, G3m, A2m and Em respectively. Polymorphism is not extensive and alleles are in strong linkage disequilibrium, usually being observed as 'established' haplotypic combinations. These haplotype associations can be characteristic for certain populations. There have been several reports of associations between Gm allotypes and autoimmune diseases. Data are consistent with there being an interaction or additive effect between Gm and HLA types to give increased levels of susceptibility.

2.6.2 α-1 antitrypsin (α1-AT)

α1-AT inhibits most serine proteases. Its prime physiological function is the inhibition of neutrophil elastase which is capable of degrading elastin and collagen. The gene is polymorphic with the M variant being most frequent. The rare allele Z is associated with α1-AT plasma deficiency and homozygotes are prone to developing emphysema. Associations between Z and S alleles and RA have been described although results are conflicting. The association between RA and the Z allele is seen most strongly in those patients with obstructive airways disease. It has also been suggested that reduced levels of this inhibitor may be related to more extensive erosions of articular cartilage in RA.

2.6.3 T cell receptor genes

T cells are central to the development of autoimmunity in that they regulate both B cell responses and cell mediated damage. As an immune response depends on the recognition of a complex of antigen and self MHC by a T cell receptor (TCR), it is a reasonable assumption that genes encoding the TCR specificity will contribute towards autoimmune susceptibility.

Two types of TCR are found, one comprising α/β chains, the other γ/δ chains. The majority of both CD4-positive cells and CD8-positive cells bear α/β TCR. The α/β TCR chains are covalently bound whereas the γ/δ TCR chains are non-covalently bound. The genes for α and δ chains are encoded on chromosome 14. The genes for β and γ chains are located on chromosome 7. Each chain is composed of a variable and a constant region. TCR variable regions are composed by different genes for the variable (V) joining (J) and diversity (D) segments for β and δ chains and V and J segments for α and γ chains. Extensive families and subfamilies of these TCR genes are present (grouped according to the degree of sequence homology between genes) in germline DNA. During T cell development and maturation in the thymus, these genes somatically rearrange into stable TCR genes. Although TCR genes belong to the immunoglobulin superfamily genes, they differ in that they do not undergo somatic mutation or isotype switching.

The analysis of TCR repertoires and TCR gene usage with respect to autoimmune disease is in its infancy. However, there is already sufficient evidence to suggest that this will contribute significantly to our understanding of autoimmunity. Several population based studies have demonstrated associations between diseases and germline-encoded TCR genes by RFLP analysis. These associations are with polymorphisms at the germline level. A more important question is whether disease susceptibility is associated with any specific TCR rearrangement or restricted usage. It is difficult to analyze clonality of *in vitro* T cell responses and TCR expression has to be measured. TCR usage for the major gene families can be measured at the cell surface level by flow cytometry using panels of monoclonal antibodies specific for TCR gene families. Studies at the molecular level to ascertain TCR rearrangement in clonal cell responses may now advance by using 'anchored PCR' (Chapter 8). Recently it has been discovered that polymorphism also exists at the level of individual TCR V region genes.

2.7 Conclusion

The evidence for a genetic component to autoimmune susceptibility is compelling although environmental factors are clearly also important. Autoimmune diseases are polygenic and present significant problems with respect to analysis and identification of susceptibility genes. These problems and the analytical approaches taken are discussed. Associations seen between HLA antigens and autoimmune diseases have gone part of the way towards identifying genetic susceptibility factors and a number of explanations have been put forward. HLA can only explain, at best, half of the genetic susceptibility in autoimmunity and the main thrust of research is moving towards the identification of non-HLA encoded susceptibility genes.

Further reading

Arnett, F.C., Goldstein, R., Duvic, M. and Reveille, J.D. (1988) Major histocompatibility complex genes in systemic lupus erythematosus, Sjögren's Syndrome and polymyositis. *Am. J. Med.,* **85** (6A), 38.

Benjamin, R. and Parham, P. (1990) Guilt by association: HLA-B27 and ankylosing spondylitis. *Immunol. Today,* **11**, 137.

Crumpton, M.J. (1987) HLA in medicine. Br. Med. Bull. **43**, 1.

Davies, K.E. and Read, A.P. (1988) *Molecular Basis of Inherited Disease.* (D. Rickwood and D. Male, eds). IRL Press, Oxford.

Demaine, A.G., Banga, J.P. and McGregor, A.M. (1990) *The Molecular Biology of Autoimmune Disease.* Nato ASI series H: Cell Biology, Volume 38. Springer-Verlag, Berlin.

Erlich, H.A. (1989) *PCR Technology – Principles and Applications for DNA Amplification.* Macmillan, New York.

Gregersen, P.K., Silner, J. and Winchester, R.J. (1987) The Shared Epitope hypothesis. *Arthritis Rheum.,* **30**, 1025.

Hansen, J.A. and Nelson, J.L. (1990) Autoimmune diseases and HLA. *Crit. Rev. Immunol.,* **10**, 307.

Nepom, G.T. and Erlich, H. (1991) MHC Class II molecules and autoimmunity. *Ann. Rev. Immunol.,* **9**, 493.

Tiwari, J.L. and Terasaki, P.I. (1985) *HLA and Disease Associations.* Springer-Verlag, New York.

Todd, J.A., Acha-Orbeo, H., Bell, J.I. *et al.* (1988) A molecular basis for MHC class II associated autoimmunity. *Science,* **240**, 1003.

Trowsdale, J., Ragoussis, J., and Campbell, R.D. (1991) Map of the human MHC. *Immunol. Today,* **12**, 443.

3
THE NATURE OF AUTO-ANTIGENS

3.1 Auto-antigens

At a conservative estimate there are at least 10 000 cellular components which theoretically could be recognized by the immune response and act as auto-antigens. It is therefore surprising that less than 100 have been accredited as acting as auto-antigens. This figure may increase as it is realized that more diseases have an autoimmune component. However, the question remains as to whether only certain self proteins can ever act as auto-antigens and, if so, what distinguishes them from components which cannot.

The distribution and nature of the auto-antigen largely dictates the autoimmune pathology. A freely available ubiquitous antigen favors the formation of immune complexes together with complications due to their precipitation and deposition in tissue. When an antigen is confined to a particular organ, the pathology is usually restricted to that tissue or those body systems which that organ influences. A receptor acting as an auto-antigen could have its functional ability altered either by increased activity or by inactivation.

The nature of the auto-antigen may influence whether cell-mediated (T cell) or antibody-mediated (B cell) aspects of the immune response are favored, as T cell receptors and antibodies tend to recognize different structures within antigens. Thus for some auto-antigens, a predominantly T-cell mediated disease may result, whereas with others antibody-mediated disease may be favored.

3.1.1 Characterization of auto-antigens

The auto-antigen is poorly characterized for the majority of autoimmune diseases. Considerable effort has been directed towards characterizing auto-antibodies and assessing their pathological role. In contrast, most auto-antigens have only been localized to the tissue or cells where they are present. Our understanding and, consequently, the treatment of any AD rests in part on elucidating both the etiology and pathology of the condition. It is therefore of paramount importance to consider every aspect, including the fine structure of the antigen provoking the autoimmune response.

Auto-antigens are usually complicated structures, composed of a number of different antigenic sites or epitopes which can be recognized by antibodies (B cell epitopes), T cell receptors (T cell epitopes) or by both. These epitopes may be linear

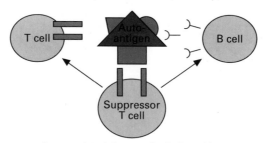

Linear or three-dimensional epitopes
on auto-antigen may be recognized by
T-cell receptors or B cells (antibody)

Auto-antigenicity may be induced by:
mutation
viruses
chemical (drug modification)
cross-reactivity (sequence homology)

Figure 3.1: *Recognition of auto-antigens.*

(continuous) amino acid sequences within the molecule; or they may be discontinuous and represent the tertiary or three-dimensional shape of the protein.

Characterization of an auto-antigen should reveal (*Figure 3.1*):

(1) whether some epitopes within the auto-antigen are more immunogenic than others; whether the auto-antigen is the site to which the pathological autoreactive response is usually directed, and whether this response is T or B cell mediated;

(2) the presence of epitopes which can induce suppressor cell function and whether this can be used to modulate the immune response;

(3) whether there is any evidence for shared antigenic structure or sequence homology at the amino acid level between self epitopes and those of infectious pathogens. This could suggest a potential trigger for the initiation of the disease process and indicate a possible treatment to remove the 'root' cause;

(4) whether the antigenic structure has been altered in any way, either at the protein level by chemical modification or at the DNA level by mutation, deletion or alternative gene splicing;

(5) whether the self-antigen involved in the disease is restricted to any one particular isotype or polymorphism.

The process of auto-antigen characterization has been hampered by difficulties in obtaining sufficient quantities of pure antigen. These are now being overcome by the gradual identification of genes encoding auto-antigens and through recombinant DNA technology whereby large quantities of pure antigen can be made.

3.1.2 Methods used to characterize auto-antigens

The principal methods used to characterize auto-antigens are summarized in *Table 3.1*. These methods are directed either at the protein or the DNA level, although some apply to both genes and their expressed products. A suggested route for characterizing an auto-antigen is depicted in *Figure 3.2*. The first step is to identify its tissue distribution. This is largely achieved by auto-antibody targeting, using indirect immunofluorescence,

Table 3.1: *Characterization of auto-antigens*

Protein level	DNA level
Tissue localization and distribution (auto-antibody) targeting-immunofluorescence, antibody–enzyme linked histology, autoradiography	Gene cloning cDNA libraries
Purification of antigen by biochemical techniques	Screening with oligonucleotide probes
Monoclonal antibody production	Expression libraries screened with monoclonal or auto-antibodies
Purification of antigen by affinity chromatography (antibody–antigen interaction)	DNA sequencing
Peptide mapping	Production of recombinant antigen
Amino acid sequencing	Chromosome localization by *in situ* hybridization
X-ray crystallography	Site-directed mutagenesis studies
Nuclear magnetic resonance	Transfection and expression studies (flow cytometry and T cell clone assays)
Immunoprecipitation studies, Western blotting of whole antigen or antigen fragments	cDNA sub-library screening following restriction enzyme digestion
2D/1D gel electrophoresis and iso-electric focusing	
Epitope mapping studies using overlapping sequential short synthetic peptides. Identification of B cell epitopes by antibody (ELISA methods) and T cell epitopes by T cell clones	

antibody-conjugated enzyme histology or autoradiography. A range of biochemical and protein chemistry techniques can be used to purify the auto-antigen and to provide a source of antigen for immunization, production and screening of monoclonal antibodies.

Alternatively, whole or fragmented antigen (cleaved by enzyme digestion or cyanogen bromide treatment) may be studied by a range of techniques such as Western blotting or iso-electric focusing. By examining the reactivity of patients' sera with antigen resolved in this way, it may be possible to identify disease-specific bands, corresponding to auto-antibodies recognizing epitopes of the auto-antigen. Such bands can be cut out from preparative gels and used to immunize animals in order to generate polyclonal or monoclonal antibodies. These antibodies are then tested against sections of the original tissue by immunofluorescence to check that they display the same pattern as the original sera from patients. Western blotting is repeated to confirm that the antisera only recognize one band. Once a monoclonal antibody has been raised it can be used to purify antigen preparations further by affinity chromatography. Pure auto-antigen can be characterized by peptide mapping or amino acid sequencing. X-ray crystallography and nuclear magnetic resonance are now being used to reveal the three-dimensional structures of molecules.

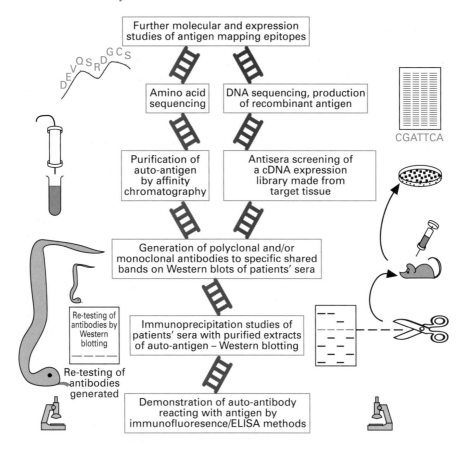

Figure 3.2: *Suggested route for characterization of auto-antigen.*

Auto-antigen characterization by molecular biology involves cloning the gene encoding its structure. Messenger RNA (mRNA) extracted from cells, originates from the coding regions of genes being actively transcribed. Complementary DNA (cDNA) can be made from mRNA using the enzyme reverse transcriptase. This procedure is outlined in *Figure 3.3*. cDNA is made from mRNA templates using an oligo(dT) primer, reverse transcriptase and nucleotide triphosphates (dNTPs). RNase can then be used to produce nicks in the mRNA strand of the mRNA/cDNA hybrid. *E. coli* DNA polymerase is used to synthesize second-strand cDNA utilizing the nicked RNA as a primer. T4 DNA polymerase is used to remove any small remaining 3' overhangs from the first-strand cDNA. cDNA can be cloned into bacteria to produce a cDNA library. These libraries can be screened in two ways. If the partial amino acid sequence of the purified protein is known, an oligonucleotide probe can be constructed which can be used for screening. A drawback of this method is that the protein has to be both known and sequenced; furthermore, there is redundancy within the triplet code for certain amino acids, giving several possibilities for the cDNA sequence. A second approach is to use a vector such as phage λgt11 to make a protein expression library which can then be screened with a relevant monoclonal antibody or with auto-antibodies from patients (*Figure 3.4*). The advantages of this approach are that the protein does not have to be purified or sequenced, and that previously unidentified auto-antigens may be picked out.

Positive clones expressing the auto-antigen can be grown up and the putative gene cut out with restriction enzymes. This gene can then be sequenced or put into an *in vitro* expression system and retested with auto-antibody. If *in vitro* expression is used it is important to realize that the protein will not be glycosylated.

Several avenues can be followed once a gene has been identified and sequenced. First, large quantities of pure recombinant antigen can be prepared from bacterial cultures. Secondly, the chromosome on which the gene is encoded can be located, together with the gene's approximate position, by using a radiolabeled cDNA oligonucleotide probe and *in situ* hybridization studies of chromosome spreads. Thirdly, the gene can be manipulated by site-directed mutagenesis. This method, first described in 1982, enables a predetermined change in any DNA sequence to be made. Various methods are available, all of which use short synthetic oligonucleotide primers. By constructing a primer that mismatches for a certain base and by following strand selection methods it is possible to substitute an amino acid in the desired position. Mutagenized genes can then be transfected and expressed in a variety of systems for further analysis at the protein level. Fourthly, the gene can be transfected into eukaryotic cells such as mouse L fibroblasts. These cells are thymidine kinase deficient and have to be maintained in supplemented medium. The auto-antigen gene

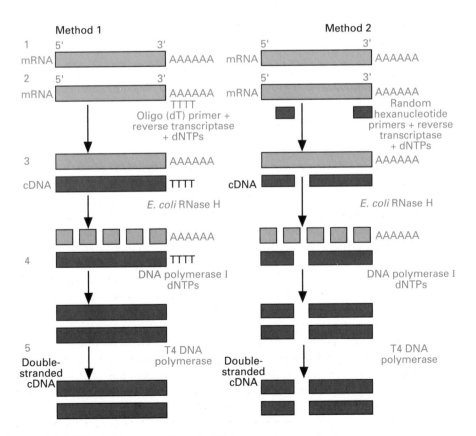

Figure 3.3: *Methods for preparation of cDNA.*

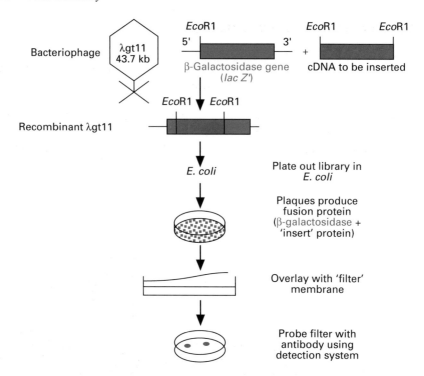

Figure 3.4: *cDNA libraries using λgt11 expression vector.*

is coupled to the thymidine kinase gene and then transfected. Only the positively transfected fibroblasts will grow in selective culture medium. Transfectants can be used for monoclonal immunization, for antibody analysis using such methods as flow cytometry, or in T cell studies as targets for T cell clones.

Further investigation of specific epitopes contained within the auto-antigen can be achieved by making a cDNA sub-library of the cloned gene. The cDNA can be cut into fragments with restriction enzymes and put into a suitable expression vector. The library can then be probed with a monoclonal antibody and the DNA inserts in positive clones can be sequenced. Thus the epitope can be narrowed down to a specific part of the whole gene sequence.

Epitope mapping has been developed recently (*Figure 3.5*). Once the amino acid sequence is known (or deduced from the DNA sequence) short overlapping peptides (usually 8 or 10 amino acids long) can be synthesized covering the whole length of the antigen sequence. These peptides can then be probed by monoclonal antibodies or by auto-antibodies using ELISA techniques. Antibody binding indicates the amino acid sequence of the B cell epitope recognized. It is very expensive to make perhaps hundreds of overlapping peptides although peptides can now be synthesized relatively cheaply on derivitized plastic pins. Once an epitope has been identified, re-synthesis of peptides where each amino acid is in turn substituted for others will reveal which amino acids are critical for antibody recognition. Such data are also useful for computer-aided molecular modelling of the epitope's three-dimensional structure. T cell epitopes can be identified by similar methods. The short overlapping peptides are put into free solution and tested with T cell clones which have been raised against the complete auto-antigen molecule.

3.1.3 Some examples of auto-antigens

It is beyond the scope of this book to review the characterization of different auto-antigens in fine detail. However, a brief summary of a limited number is given to illustrate the type of information which can be gained (*Table 3.2*).

Thyroglobulin (TG). TG is a homodimeric glycosylated iodoprotein (2×330 kd) with a sedimentation coefficient of 19S. The human TG gene is located on the long arm of chromosome 8 and comprises 42 exons. Cloning and sequencing of human and bovine

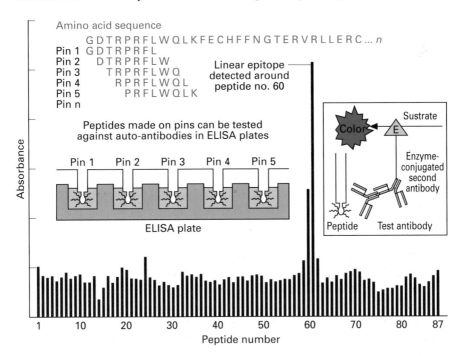

Figure 3.5: *Epitope mapping.*

TG cDNA have provided a detailed picture of the protein's primary structure. The TG polypeptide chain is 2748 residues long and can be sub-divided into four domains: A, B, C and D. The A, B and C domains each contain their own repetitive sequence motifs. The D domain, accounting for the last 600 residues, has no repetitive sequences and internal homology. The immunogenicity of TG is considerably influenced by post-translational modification and iodination. Highly iodinated TG seems to be a more potent antigenic target and high-iodine containing diets in animal models of thyroiditis potentiate the disease.

There is some sequence homology between the D domain of TG and the whole acetylcholinesterase molecule from the fish *Torpedo california* suggesting that these proteins may have a common ancestry and exhibit conserved three-dimensional characteristics. Immunological cross-reactivity between TG and the acetylcholinesterase of eye muscles may play a role in the pathology of Grave's ophthalmopathy (Section 5.3.1). Circumstantial evidence for shared epitopes between these molecules has been

Table 3.2: Examples of auto-antigens

Auto-antigen	Principal associated conditions	Physical characteristics of antigen
Thyroglobulin (TG)	Grave's Disease Hashimoto's thyroiditis	Glycosylated iodoprotein homodimer. Four domains to antigen, 2×330 kd. Encoded on chromosome 8.
Thyroid peroxidase (TPO) (thyroid microsomal antigen)	Grave's Disease Hashimoto's thyroiditis	Bound to plasma membrane of thyroid follicular cells. Two molecular forms, 105 kd and 110 kd. Encoded on chromosome 2.
Acetylcholine receptor(AChR)	Myasthenia gravis	Role in neuromuscular transmission. Made up of 5 units: 2α, β, γ, δ.
Extractable nuclear antigen SS-B/La	Primary Sjögren's Syndrome	Associated with precursors of RNA polymerase. 47 kd. Homology with retroviral gag protein.

demonstrated by the isolation of TG clones from a λgt11 library with rabbit anti-acetylcholinesterase antibody. Sequence homology also exists between domain A of TG and the invariant chain of class II MHC molecules which is involved in intracellular movement of molecules and antigen processing. This suggests that the A domain of TG may be important in its transfer to specific intracellular sites.

Considerable effort has gone into the mapping of epitopes within the TG molecule. Screening of λgt11 cDNA libraries containing cDNA inserts of human thyroid, followed by sequencing of clones detected by antisera, has led to the identification of ten non-overlapping epitope bearing fragments. In addition, deletion mutants have been produced by sequentially removing stretches of bases from the 3' ends of cDNAs by enzymatic cleavage, without changing the translational frame for the gene. After insertion of such mutants into an expression system, the recombinant proteins are evaluated for auto-epitopes by testing with patients' sera.

*Thyroid peroxidase (TPO).*TPO is a glycosylated protein, bound to the plasma membrane of thyroid follicular cells, with its active enzymatic domain facing the colloid space. The TPO gene is on chromosome 2. TPO can be isolated in two molecular forms, 105 kd and 110 kd. TPO has been cloned and sequenced giving the primary structure of the protein. Two cDNAs, differing by 171 nucleotides, have been identified, which result from alternative gene splicing. Hydrophobicity profiles indicate that TPO is anchored in the cell membrane by a segment close to its carboxy terminus. The extracellular domain of the molecule has 42% sequence homology with myeloperoxidase suggesting a common ancestry. Screening of λgt11 cDNA libraries with auto-antibodies has demonstrated unequivocally that thyroid microsomal antigen and TPO are the same molecule. Several auto-antigenic sites have been delineated on TPO to which pathogenic auto-antibodies are directed. By using the polymerase chain reaction to amplify segments of the TPO sequence, followed by expression as recombinant fusion proteins, further epitopes have been identified.

*Acetylcholine receptor (AChR).*The disease myasthenia gravis (MG) is due to the binding of auto-antibodies to the nicotinic acetylcholine receptor (AChR). This results in a defect in neuromuscular transmission (Section 6.5.1). The human AChR consists of two α, one β, one γ and one δ sub-units. Each one traverses the cell membrane at least four times. Two-thirds of MG patients have auto-antibodies to an extracellular area of the AChR α sub-unit, named the main immunogenetic region. Through epitope mapping studies, this region has been located between residues 67 and 76 of the α sub-unit. Antibodies to this region can passively transfer experimental MG in rats. By the substitution of amino acids in synthetic peptides corresponding to the main immunogenetic region sequence, it has been concluded that residues 68 (Asn) and 71 (Asp) are vital for monoclonal antibody binding. AChR genes have been transfected into mouse fibroblast L cells and should provide a useful resource in the study of AChR–auto-antibody binding.

Extractable nuclear antigen SS-B/La. The La antigen is a small nuclear ribonucleoprotein (SnRNP) with a molecular weight of 47 kd. Antibodies to this antigen are strongly associated with primary Sjögren's Syndrome (Section 5.11). The antigen is mainly associated with the precursors of RNA polymerase transcripts, including tRNAs and virus encoded RNAs. The gene for the La protein has been cloned and recombinant antigen is available for study. Mapping of auto-epitopes within the La antigen has been performed by various methods including the production of deletion mutant La genes by the removal of bases from the 3' ends of cDNA. A number of epitopes have been identified by following this method. One epitope (amino acids 88–101) has high homology to a retroviral gag protein.

3.2 Possible environmental triggers for autoimmunity

The key question in the study of autoimmune disease is "How has the body been induced to react against itself?". Clearly the answer is multifactorial. Some patients are genetically susceptible to autoimmune disease (Chapter 2) and the ageing process is associated with a decline in the efficiency of immune surveillance leading to an increased frequency of both malignancy and of autoimmune disease. These two facets explain a propensity in some patients to produce auto-antibodies. It is possible that the auto-antibodies may occur spontaneously as part of the extensive B cell repertoire. However, it is also possible that the production of auto-antibodies is triggered by some subtle alteration in the configuration of normal tissues – the production of auto-antigens. Again this may occur spontaneously or it may be induced by external agents. Such external agents include infections, drugs, toxins, ultraviolet radiation and smoking *(Table 3.3)*. This section examines the way in which viruses and other environmental agents may induce the production of autoimmunity.

3.2.1 The role of infection in autoimmunity

Many chronic infections are associated with autoimmune phenomena. For example, patients with leprosy, syphilis or tuberculosis often have rheumatoid factors (RF)

Table 3.3: *Environmental agents which may precipitate autoimmunity*

Infections – bacterial and viral
Drugs
Toxins
Ultraviolet radiation
Smoking

---

detectable in the blood, as well as auto-antibodies directed against the thyroid gland, skeletal muscle and the adrenal gland, for example. However, the ability of modern bacteriological methods to detect organisms is such that it is unlikely that many autoimmune diseases are due to undiagnosed bacterial infections. The possibility of 'molecular mimicry' following infection may play a role in some diseases. For example, following infections with group A streptococci, patients may develop rheumatic fever. The anti-streptococcal antibodies produced by the body cross-react with antigens found in the human heart. It is also possible that heat shock proteins induced by bacterial infection may provoke autoimmune phenomena.

3.2.2 *Heat shock proteins and autoimmunity*

Heat shock proteins (HSPs), or stress proteins, are produced by prokaryotic and eukaryotic cells in response to a range of physiological insults including infection. They were thought classically to be induced by increased temperature, but a variety of stressful conditions such as anoxia and exposure to reactive oxygen species (frequently produced in inflammation) can provoke even higher levels of HSP than fever.

HSPs were originally considered to be protective: preventing the unfolding of proteins and DNA at high temperatures. However, it is now known that HSPs are present in normal unstressed cells and that they have vital 'house-keeping' roles, 'chaperoning' proteins. HSPs also act as important antigens of infectious organisms, often providing the major stimulus for an immune response (*Table 3.4*). A paradox exists in that many T cells can recognize and respond to bacterial HSPs despite a very high degree of sequence homology being conserved in HSPs, from yeast through to human cells.

All HSPs belong to a superfamily in which most are defined on the basis of their molecular mass. These families include 90 kd HSP, 70 kd HSP, 60 kd HSP ubiquitin. The 90 kd HSP complexes with the steroid receptor, preventing it from binding non-specifically to DNA. Both 70 kd HSP and 60 kd HSP members are involved in protein folding, translocation and assembly within the cell. Ubiquitin has a role in protein degradation. All of these HSPs have been implicated in autoimmunity. Increased antibody levels to HSPs have been observed in RA (65 kd HSP), ankylosing spondylitis (90 kd HSP) and SLE (ubiquitin, 70 kd HSP and 90 kd HSP). How these HSPs are involved in autoimmunity is not known. One possibility is that, although these proteins are usually hidden within the intracellular compartment, in certain situations they may be expressed on the cell surface and either trigger autoimmune responses or act as targets for auto-antibodies. The human 65 kd HSP molecule shares

Table 3.4: Heat shock proteins

Family	Major members	Function and role
Ubiquitin	Ubiquitin	Involved in protein degradation, processing of class I MHC antigens, lymphocyte homing and implicated in autoimmunity
HSP 60	HSP 65, groEL	Involved in protein folding and unfolding. These are potent antigens for many pathogens and have been implicated in autoimmunity
HSP 70	HSP 70, BiP, hsc 70, grp 78, dnak	Involved in protein folding, unfolding and translocation, also in the assembly of multimeric complexes
HSP 90	HSP 90, HSP 83	Prevents the steroid receptor binding to DNA, tyrosine kinase phosphorylation. Implicated in tumor resistance and autoimmunity

approximately 65% sequence homology with mycobacterial 65 kd HSP, suggesting that it may be a potential antigen for autoreactive T cells. Considerable *in vitro* evidence supports this conclusion and T cell clones recognizing shared epitopes between these HSPs have been prepared from normal individuals. This indicates that the normal T cell repertoire includes potentially autoreactive T cells to HSPs, which may be activated given suitable exposure to 'cross-reactive' bacterial HSPs during infection.

The best evidence for involvement of HSPs in autoimmunity is seen in RA. Experimentally induced synovitis can be provoked by immunization of rats with mycobacterial-based adjuvant and T cell lines made against HSP can passively transfer arthritis to naive animals. The 65 kd HSP is more abundant and strongly expressed on synovial lining cells in RA patients than in normal individuals. Many of the T cells responding to HSPs bear γ/δ TCRs. It has been suggested that these T cells may be directed against autologous HSPs, so as to recognize and eliminate 'stressed' host cells, perhaps during inflammation.

Two 70 kd HSP genes have recently been reported within the MHC. Whether this has relevance to HLA associations with autoimmunity is not yet known. Many new genes with unknown function have been found around HSP 70 in the MHC class III region.

3.2.3 Viruses and autoimmunity

Viruses are the strongest infective candidates for a role in the production of autoimmune diseases. Several theoretical mechanisms have been suggested by which viral infections might provoke autoimmunity: some of these have already been discussed in Section 2.5.4. The virus might alter the structure or the rate of synthesis of the host cell surface antigens. Alternatively, the virus might activate the immune system; or molecular mimicry might exist between host antigens and viral sequences. The evidence to support such theories is derived largely from experimental animals and not from humans. Adenovirus and reovirus infection in rat thyroid cells induces MHC class II antigen expression. In humans, adenovirus infection has been shown to cause the auto-antigen La (normally located within the nucleus – see Section 3.1.3) to increase in quantity and migrate from the nucleus to be expressed on the cell surface. As yet the case for virus-induced autoimmunity in man is far from proven but this remains an interesting and fruitful line of research. Retroviruses and Epstein–Barr virus are worthy of particular mention.

Retroviruses. Retroviruses all possess the enzyme reverse transcriptase, an RNA-directed DNA polymerase. At the time of infection this enzyme catalyzes synthesis of a DNA 'provirus' from the virion RNA and this provirus becomes incorporated into the chromosomal DNA of the host. The genomes of most vertebrates contain numerous retroviral sequences most of which are not infectious. These endogenous sequences are transcribed and translated in many host tissues. Mouse strains which are susceptible to autoimmune diseases have increased expression of RNA coding for a full-length type C retrovirus. This is vertically transmitted from mother to offspring. It has been shown that inhibition of synthesis of the endogenous retroviral envelope proteins results in lymphocyte stimulation. This suggests that the endogenous retroviral envelope proteins may be involved in a negative feedback circuit.

Retroviruses can be sub-divided into three families: the oncovirinae, the lentivirinae and the spumavirinae. The lentiviruses include the caprine arthritis encephalitis virus, which produces a naturally occurring arthritis resembling RA in sheep and goats. Until 1980 no human retrovirus had been described. However, four major classes of human retroviruses have now been discovered. The human T cell lymphotrophic viruses are oncoviruses associated with adult T cell leukemia-lymphoma and T cell hairy cell leukemia. Similar viruses have been implicated as the cause of multiple sclerosis and tropical spastic paraparesis but the case is not fully proven. Human lentiviruses include the human immunodeficiency virus (HIV) which is responsible for the acquired immunodeficiency syndrome (AIDS) (see below). A spumavirus may be the cause of de Quervain's thyroiditis.

In HIV infection the virus binds to the CD4 antigen receptor site. This is followed by cell lysis and CD4 lymphopenia. HIV may also infect macrophages, B cells already infected with Epstein–Barr virus (see below) and certain other T cells. Abnormalities in the activation and regulation of B cells occur and patients develop hypergammaglobulinemia. Joint pains associated with dry eyes, dry mouth and parotid enlargement (i.e. Sjögren's Syndrome (SS) – Section 5.11) have been described in patients with HIV infection. The lymphocytes infiltrating the parotid are predominantly CD8-positive as opposed to the CD4-positive cells seen in classical SS. Patients with this HIV-associated syndrome often have circulating RF and antinuclear antibodies but rarely anti-Ro or anti-La. Patients with HIV infection may show other autoimmune phenomena: polymyositis, SLE, autoimmune thrombocytopenia and vasculitis.

Epstein–Barr virus. The Epstein–Barr virus (EBV) is a lymphotropic herpes virus originally isolated from an African Burkitt's lymphoma cell line. Within the lymphoid system the virus only infects B cells and causes polyclonal B cell activation. The virus in EBV is ubiquitous. The exact pattern of infection is related to geographic and socioeconomic status. In underdeveloped countries 90% of children are infected by the age of five. In the developed countries infection occurs most commonly in the teenage years producing the disease called infectious mononucleosis (glandular fever). Like all herpes viruses, EBV has the property of viral latency. In normal individuals 1 in 100 000 B lymphocytes carry the virus indefinitely post-infection. The virus is thought to replicate in the salivary glands. A number of cell systems are important in controlling EBV infection. These include a T-cell dependent γ-interferon-mediated suppressor activity and cytotoxic T cells which kill EBV infected cells.

Burkitt's lymphoma (a form of non-Hodgkin's lymphoma endemic in Africa) is closely associated with EBV and there is serological evidence of inadequate virus control long before the tumor appears. EBV is also associated with other non-Hodgkin's lymphomas, especially those associated with post-transplantation immunosuppression and congenital immunodeficiency states.

Epstein–Barr nuclear antigen is a marker of cells containing the EB viral genome. It can be detected by immunofluorescence. A high percentage of RA patients have antibodies to another EBV nuclear antigen called RANA. When this phenomenon was first described it was thought to be unique to RA and so EBV was postulated as the cause of RA. However, RANA has now been demonstrated in normal individuals. A defective T cell response to EBV-infected B cells has also been described in RA, scleroderma and SS. EBV is found in salivary gland cells and is a major candidate as a cause of SS.

3.2.4 Superantigens and autoimmunity

Superantigens (SAs) are proteins which have the capacity to stimulate a large fraction of T cells expressing particular TCR Vβ sequences. This growing family of antigens includes staphylococcal enterotoxins ($A, B, C_1, C_2, C_3, D, E$), streptococcal M protein and an, as yet, unidentified product of *Mycoplasma arthritidis*.

Approximately 1 in 5 to 1 in 50 T cells respond to these antigens, whereas T cells responding clonally to an antigen are in the order of 1:10 000 to 1:100 000. SAs can often activate T cells at picomolar concentrations and induce the release of large amounts of IL-2, IFN-γ and tumor necrosis factor (TNF). MHC class II molecules are high affinity receptors for SAs and binding is required for efficient interaction with the TCR. Binding of SA to class II does not appear to be in the peptide binding groove nor does it require any antigen processing (*Figure 3.6*). Each SA activates a specific panel of T cells depending on the TCR Vβ sequence (*Table 3.5*). All T cells with these sequences appear to be activated irrespective of whether they are CD4, CD8, memory or naive cells. The activation of T cells by SA can lead to the production of cytotoxic T cells against MHC class II positive antigen-presenting cells.

A second type of SA mimics many of the bacterial SAs and may have fundamental importance in autoimmune susceptibility. These are endogenous 'self-SAs' encoded by retroviruses and, as yet, they have only been characterized in mice. Like other retroviruses, those encoding SAs may be inherited via the genome or transmitted via the milk. The minor lymphocyte stimulating system in the mouse has been shown to be due to retroviral sequences. The presence of a particular self-SA results in the activation of T cells bearing particular Vβ elements. These cells will be deleted in the thymus before maturation in order to maintain non-responsiveness or tolerance to self-SAs. Thus the deletion of T cells expressing a particular Vβ is indicative of the

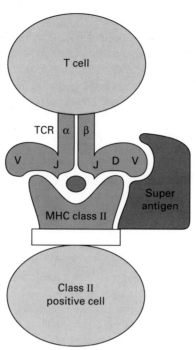

Figure 3.6: Binding of superantigens.

presence of the corresponding self-SA.

It seems unlikely that this phenomenon is restricted to mice. If present in the human it would represent a major element in the shaping of the T cell repertoire and the selection of Vβ genes. This would result in potential 'holes' in the T cell repertoire and might have important implications for recognition of auto-antigens and the development of AD.

Table 3.5: Superantigen–Vβ interactions

Foreign superantigens	Human Vβ specificity
Staphylococcal enterotoxin	
A	?
B	Vβ3, 12, 14, 15, 17, 20
C₁	Vβ12
C₂	Vβ12, 13, 14, 15, 17, 20
C₃	Vβ5, 12
D	Vβ5, 12
E	Vβ5.1, 6.1–6.3, 8, 18
Toxic shock syndrome – T1	Vβ2
Exfoliating toxins A,B	Vβ2
Mycoplasma arthritidis supernatant	Vβ?
Endogenous superantigens	
? Retroviruses	Vβ?

3.2.5 Other environmental factors and autoimmunity

It is possible that ubiquitous environmental agents such as common constituents of the diet play an important role in triggering certain ADs. Such a case would be very hard to prove. There are a number of instances where environmental agents have been implicated directly in AD. Drugs have been implicated in a number of ADs, in particular SLE, myasthenia gravis and idiopathic thrombocytopenic purpura (ITP). Penicillamine has been described as causing a variety of ADs including myasthenia, ITP, scleroderma, myositis and pemphigus.

Environmental toxins, especially silicon and vinyl chloride have been associated with scleroderma. Scleroderma is weakly associated with HLA-DR5, -DR3 and -B8. Patients developing vinyl chloride disease have an increased frequency of DR5. Most workers with DR5 exposed to vinyl chloride develop the disease. However, those B8, DR3 workers who develop the disease have a very severe form. Thus this disease illustrates the interaction between a disease susceptibility gene, a disease severity gene, and a known environmental trigger. It has also been suggested that cases of scleroderma may be found in clusters around airports and that aircraft fuel might be an environmental trigger.

Ultraviolet radiation may trigger exacerbations of SLE. Cigarette smoking is associated with the lung complications of Goodpasture's Syndrome. The search for such agents is continuing and much depends on the astuteness of clinicians and patient groups in picking up possible leads.

3.2.6 Hormonal factors and autoimmunity

The sex hormones (estrogen, progesterone and testosterone) can all profoundly influence the functioning of the immune system. Generally speaking, immune tolerance can be induced more easily in males, and females reject transplants and tumors more effectively. Compared to men, women have higher immunoglobulin levels, increased antibody production after immunization and decreased susceptibility to certain infections. Yet women are able to maintain the 9 month gestation of a fetus which is genetically dissimilar to themselves. These differences appear to be due to hormonal rather than chromosomal differences between the sexes as castration leads to a 'feminizing' of the immune system in males.

Most ADs are more common in women than men (Section 5.2). A higher prevalence of AD is also seen in Klinefelter's Syndrome (karyotype XXY). Some observations in RA illustrate the complex relationship between hormone status and autoimmunity. RA is rare before puberty. In the pre-menopausal years the female to male ratio is greater than in the post-menopausal years when it approaches unity. The oral contraceptive pill appears to lower the risk of developing RA and the disease often goes into remission during pregnancy. Yet post-partum flares in disease activity are common. Similarly, disease onset during pregnancy is rare.

Animal studies also implicate sex hormones in autoimmunity. In two mouse models of SLE, female hormones accelerate the disease process and the female mice die before the males. However, in the BXSB mouse, males develop the disease much earlier than the females. In this strain the male disadvantage is mediated by an 'accelerating gene' on the Y chromosome rather than by hormones.

Sex hormones act via their different surface receptors directly on T cells, especially CD8-positive cells. Estrogens can increase levels of antibody production by inhibiting T suppressor activity. Progesterone, on the other hand, increases T suppressor function. In animal models of experimentally induced arthritis, estrogens may improve the arthritis. However, the effect varies according to the inducing agent and species used. Increased levels of estrogen in humans occur in adolescence, at the menarche and in pregnancy. In the puerperium there is a drastic fall in estrogen but an even sharper fall in progesterone leading to an estrogen excess.

Thus it is clear that hormones can influence the immune system and play a part in the higher frequency of autoimmunity in females. However, understanding of their role is still incomplete and attempts to modulate the hormonal milieu in established human AD have been inconclusive.

3.3 Conclusion

In autoimmunity the body's immune system reacts against some of its own components. We have seen in Chapter 2 that some patients are genetically susceptible to AD. Yet even in these individuals some event must trigger the development of AD. One of the earliest events in this process seems to be the recognition of auto-antigens. Characterization of those parts of the body which can act as auto-antigens and comparing the structure and function of these antigens in healthy and diseased individuals will show whether a change has occurred. Possible triggers of such changes must be sought in the environment. They are likely to be infectious agents or their consequences, and physical or chemical stimuli.

Further reading

Demaine, A.G., Banga, J.P. and McGregor, A.M. (1990) *The Molecular Biology of Autoimmune Disease*. NATO ASI series H, Cell Biology, Volume 38. Springer–Verlag, Berlin.

Geysen, H.M., Rodda, S.J., Mason, T.J., Tribbick, G. and Schoofs, P.G. (1987) Strategies for epitope analysis using peptide synthesis. *J. Immunol. Methods*, **102**, 259.

Herman, A., Kappler, J.W., Marrack, P. and Pullen, A.M. (1991) Superantigens: mechanisms of T-cell stimulation and role in immune responses. *Ann. Rev. Immunol.*, **9**, 745.

Janeway, C. (1991) MIS: Makes a little sense. *Nature*, **349**, 459.

Kaufmann, S.H.E. (1990) Heat shock proteins and the immune response. *Immunol. Today*, **11**, 129.

Kimura, S., Kotani, T., McBride, O.W., Umeki, K., Hirai, K., Nakayama, T. and Ohtaki, S. (1987) Human thyroid peroxidase; complete cDNA and protein sequence, chromosome mapping, and identification of two alternatively spliced mRNAs. *Proc. Natl Acad. Sci. USA*, **84**, 5555.

Kohsaka, H., Yamamoto, K., Fujii, H., Miura, H., Miyasaka, N., Nishioka, K. and Miyamoto, Y. (1990) Fine epitope mapping of the human SSB/La protein. *J. Clin. Invest.*, **85**, 1566.

Rapoport, B., Hirayu, H., Seto, P. and Magnusson, R.P. (1987) Molecular cloning of antigens to thyroid autoantibodies using the expression vector lambda gt11. *Acta Endocrinol.*, **281** *Suppl.*, 139.

4

THE CONSEQUENCES OF AUTOIMMUNITY AT CELLULAR AND HUMORAL LEVELS

It is artificial to divide the cellular and humoral components of autoimmunity since the two are, of course, part of the same response. Nevertheless it is convenient to consider in turn the processes mediated by lymphocytic infiltration and those mediated by auto-antibodies.

4.1 T cells in autoimmunity

T cells are central to the generation of an immune response regardless of whether this is to a foreign or a self-antigen. Recognition of antigen by T cells through their TCRs can trigger a series of events which may ultimately result in cytotoxic T cell production and antibody production by B cells. These effects, and more, are largely mediated through the action of cytokines (*Figure 4.1*). T cell proliferation is largely antigen driven and the α/β TCRs of CD4 helper T cells usually recognize antigen only if it has been processed and presented by antigen-presenting cells (APCs) expressing autologous class II MHC molecules (Section 2.5.2).

Recognition of antigen by TCRs only takes place by contact either of helper T cells and APCs, or of cytotoxic T cells and target cells. A set of accessory molecules (the cell-surface glycoproteins CD4, CD8, CD2 and the lymphocyte functional antigen, LFA-1) play a critical role in cell–cell contact. This may be in establishing cell adhesion, stabilizing TCR/antigen binding and giving either positive or negative signals which assist in the early phases of T cell activation.

4.1.1 Accessory and adhesion molecules

As discussed in Chapter 2, a relationship exists, although not absolute, between the expression of CD4 or CD8 and T cell recognition of antigen presented by class II and class I MHC molecules respectively. It has been suggested that CD4 and CD8 may serve as additional recognition elements and bind to monomorphic regions of class II and class I MHC. Both CD2 and LFA-1 bind to ligands (LFA-3 and ICAM-1, respectively) on the surface of target cells or APCs. CD2 and LFA-1 act in concert with the TCR for T cell activation. CD2 is also important in T cell ontogeny and thymic education (Section 1.3.1). LFA-1 is found not only on T cells but also on the surface of B cells, monocytes, activated macrophages and neutrophils. LFA-1 belongs to a family of cell adhesion molecules known as intergrins. The role of adhesion molecules

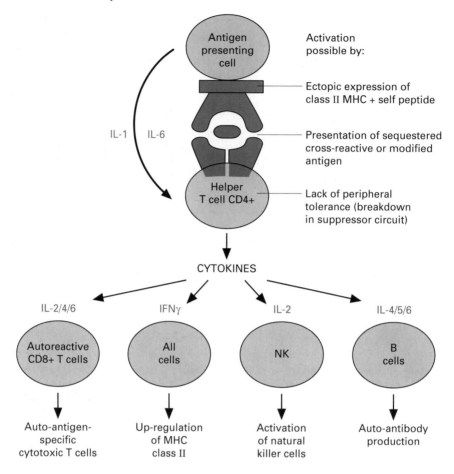

Figure 4.1: *The central role of T cells in generating an immune response.*

in autoimmunity is unclear although there are reports of increased cell surface expression in some conditions.

4.1.2 T cell recognition and activation

Contact between T cells and APCs, and between T and B cells, is necessary for the optimal functioning of the immune response. Similarly, cytolytic activity is dependent on contact between T cells and their targets. The initial contact does not primarily require an interaction between the TCR and its target antigen, but is non-specifically mediated via LFA-1 and CD2. The adhesion between LFA-1 and ICAM-1 is magnesium-ion dependent, whereas that between CD2 and LFA-3 is not. Most studies to investigate this adhesion phase have used cytotoxic T cells and it is not known if the same holds true for helper T cells. However, it is thought that non-specific adhesion is important in T cell activation by APCs. The CD2 and LFA-1 adhesion pathways may also be important in T/B cell co-operation in antibody production.

Following initial adhesion, T cells can be activated as a consequence of an antigen

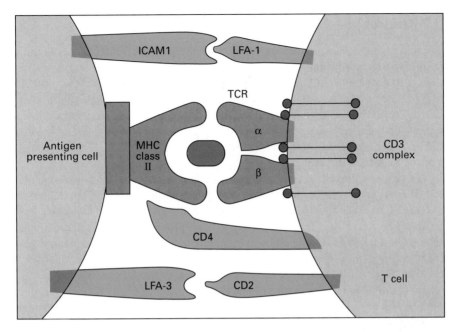

Figure 4.2: *Cell surface molecules involved in APC–T-cell interaction and activation.*

being presented to, and binding with the TCR–CD3 complex. The TCR endows specificity to this activation. The CD3 component chains have long intracellular domains which interact with cytoplasmic proteins involved in signal transduction and amplification. The cell surface structures involved in APC–T-cell interactions are represented in *Figure 4.2*.

Early in T cell activation there is a rise in intracellular calcium and pH, an efflux of potassium, increased turnover of phosphoinositols and activation of protein kinase C. Although these changes are triggered by the TCR–CD3 complex, T cell activation and proliferation also requires secondary signals provided by accessory cells such as macrophages. These secondary signals are poorly understood.

4.1.3 γ/δ *T cells*

The majority of mature T cells express α/β TCR molecules on the cell surface in association with CD3. A small sub-set of T cells has now been identified which have γ/δ TCRs associated with CD3. These cells lack both the CD4 and CD8 markers. They are usually cytolytic and often have natural killer cell-like activity (Section 4.2). These γ/δ T cells proliferate in response to allogenic cells in mixed lymphocyte cultures and can lyse targets bearing the stimulating allo-antigen. Heterogeneity of γ/δ T cells has been identified using monoclonal antibodies, with one type prevalent in the peripheral blood and absent in the thymus. Another type is infrequent in peripheral blood but represents the majority of γ/δ T cells in the thymus. The latter express the CD8 antigen when cultured with IL-2. The possible role of these recently identified T cells in autoimmunity has yet to be evaluated.

4.2 Natural killer cells

Lymphocytoxic reactions which are independent of class I and II MHC recognition can be mediated by two distinct types of lymphocytes. The most common are natural killer (NK) cells which are CD3-negative, large granular lymphocytes. They do not rearrange and express TCR genes but have the characteristic cell surface markers CD16 (Fc γRIII – the low affinity receptor for the IgG Fc) and NKH-1 (Leu 19). A second cell type displaying similar cytotoxicity consists of a small sub-population of CD3-positive lymphocytes which express either the α/β or γ/δ TCR. These are usually referred to as 'NK-like' cells.

NK cells are thought to arise principally in the bone marrow. They are present in considerable numbers in the peripheral blood, spleen and peritoneum. The relationship of NK cells to CD3-positive T cells is unclear, although it is thought that they have separate lineages. NK cells may represent a more 'primitive' type of cell providing a less discriminatory but highly efficient immunity to genetically unrelated target cells or transformed (virally or malignant) cells. It has been suggested that the cytotoxic T cell responses with MHC-restricted killing have evolved from NK cells while retaining the functional properties of NK cells.

The precise nature of target cell recognition by NK cells is unclear but is thought to result from a complex of receptor–ligand interactions such as CD2 –LFA-3 or LFA-1–ICAM-1. It is interesting to note that the molecules used by NK cells have been retained by T cells and function as accessory receptors required for efficient TCR-directed recognition in MHC-restricted cytotoxicity.

Lymphokine-activated killer cells (LAK) are IL-2-activated lymphocytes in either of the categories above. IL-2 will, in general, dramatically enhance the levels of all NK activity. Cytokines have a range of effects on NK cells, some acting as a 'progression factor' (IL-4) and others in the maintenance and activation of cells (IL-2, IL-3). There is also evidence that lysis by NK cells requires α-interferon and is mediated through TNF.

A role for NK cells and 'NK-like' cells in autoimmune processes is clear given the localized inflammation and production of cytokines such as IL-2. However, the relative contributions of NK cells and T cells in autoimmune processes are uncertain and may differ between conditions.

4.3 Mechanisms of cell-mediated lysis

Cytotoxic T lymphocytes (CTLs), NK cells and lymphocytes engaged in antibody-dependent cell cytotoxicity (ADCC) are thought to lyse target cells by a number of different mechanisms, some of which they hold in common. A key mediator found in these cell types is a pore-forming protein called perforin or cytolysin. This protein is located in cytoplasmic granules which are released following contact between effector and target cells. In the presence of extracellular calcium, perforin binds to the target membrane and undergoes conformation changes into tubules, resulting in irreversible damage to the target cells. Perforin affects membrane permeability causing influx of water and leakage of electrolytes resulting in death and lysis. Cytotoxic lymphocytes can recycle after they have damaged target cells and lyse further target cells. CTLs have a high resistance to self-lysis by perforin. The *in vivo* role of perforin in cytotoxicity remains unclear as most data have come from analysis of *in vitro* CTL lines. Detectable levels of perforin have been found only in spleen and peritoneal lymphocytes maintained in culture with IL-2. The perforin pathway has absolute dependence on calcium. As many CTL populations can lyse targets in the absence of calcium, this suggests that there are multiple mechanisms for cytolysis.

The DNA of some target cells undergoes fragmentation into units of 150–180 bp through the action of CTL and NK cells. Whether this endonuclease activity comes from the effector cells or is activated endogenously within the target cell as a suicide pathway is unknown. It has yet to be established whether DNA fragmentation represents the cause or the consequence of cell death.

A tumor necrosis factor/lymphotoxin-like activity has been detected in the supernatants of activated T cells and CTLs known to be effective in fragmenting target cell DNA. Serine esterase and proteoglycans have also been suggested as candidate mediators of cytotoxicity for CTLs and NK cells.

4.4 B cell responses in autoimmunity

Auto-antibodies, like ADs themselves, may be organ or non-organ specific. Auto-antibodies can be pathogenic and play a central role in disease processes. Alternatively, they can be present, have no significant pathogenic role and sometimes may even be beneficial. As discussed in Section 1.3, self-tolerance to auto-antigens at the B cell level and auto-antibody regulation is largely mediated by T cells. T cell help is only possible when the T cell recognizes the self-antigen and provides the cytokine signals necessary for B cell triggering and clonal expansion. Thus the T cell is central to most B cell responses and the production of auto-antibodies can be considered as a failure in T cell regulation. The ways by which this regulation can be bypassed were discussed in Chapter 1.

A proportion of B cells (those expressing the CD5 marker) do not need this T cell help. Furthermore, individuals may already possess the immunoglobulin genes necessary for producing some auto-antibodies.

4.4.1 CD5-positive B cells

CD5 is strongly expressed on T cells and also on a sub-set of B lymphocytes. There is some debate as to whether this is a B cell lineage or an activation marker. CD5-positive B cells are generated early in ontogeny and from then on are found mainly in the peritoneum although also in the peripheral blood. They are self-generating rather than being formed in the bone marrow.

CD5-positive B cells produce the majority of natural antibodies in the serum, many of which are directed against important bacterial antigens in the environment and also cross-react with self-antigens. However, these antibodies are not thought to be auto-aggressive and provide an early form of natural immunity to bacterial infections. Such antibodies are probably germline encoded.

Considerable interest has been shown in these B cells as increased numbers are found in a variety of human autoimmune conditions including RA, SLE, multiple sclerosis, Hashimoto's thyroiditis, Grave's Disease and Sjögren's Syndrome. These cells produce the majority of IgM rheumatoid factor in *in vitro* cultures and also other auto-antibodies of low affinity. IgM antibodies produced by CD5-positive B cells are independent of T cell control, although T cells can dramatically augment IgM responses and induce IgA and IgG antibodies. CD5-positive B cells can act as antigen presenters and may be important in the development of anti-idiotypes (Section 1.2.1). It has been suggested that CD5-positive B cells may drive some AD processes.

There is evidence that CD5 expression on B cells is under genetic control. The majority of polyclonal activators do not increase CD5 surface expression, although this can be achieved with IL-2. The activation process for CD5-positive B cells appears to be selective, which may account for their self-generation and paucity in the bone marrow. Chronic lymphocytic leukemia is due to malignant transformation of CD5-positive B cells. As a number of AD are associated with an increased risk of this leukemia (Section 7.2) this provides further evidence to link CD5-positive B cells with autoimmunity.

4.4.2 The genetic basis for auto-antibody specificity

Immunoglobulin gene rearrangements and somatic mutations occur continually throughout life and, as a consequence, auto-antibodies can potentially arise at any time. The specificity and production of auto-antibodies has two components, one largely determined genetically and the other due to antigenic selection. It is therefore of primary importance to consider whether the inherited repertoire of variable region genes influences the potential to produce specific auto-antibodies and how regulatory mechanisms prevent the expansion of self-reactive B lymphocytes.

Auto-antibodies may already be encoded as germline immunoglobulin genes and may be present in the pre-immune B cell repertoire. Alternatively, they may only arise following rearrangement and mutation. These situations are not mutually exclusive. A non-specific immune stimulus, such as graft versus host disease, can induce auto-antibody production in animals, suggesting that auto-antibody precursors exist in the germline. Whichever situation applies, long-term auto-antibody synthesis is usually antigen driven. This is indicated by the increase in antibody affinity seen over time and immunoglobulin class switching.

Auto-antibodies can be made by both CD5-positive and CD5-negative B cells. However, CD5-positive cells are in a strong idiotypic regulatory network and have limited potential for clonal expansion. Thus CD5-positive B cells give relatively limited antibody responses and produce antibodies with a predominantly 'housekeeping' role.

4.4.3 Idiotypic networks

The idiotypic network theory put forward by Jerne suggests that regulatory networks of interacting anti-idiotypic antibodies are initiated after primary antigen exposure and the generation of new antibodies by the host. Anti-idiotypic antibodies are essentially auto-antibodies and it is suggested that they may have a role in both suppression and amplification of responses. Animal studies indicate that several rounds of anti-idiotypic antibodies can be generated after an initial antibody response. Any response to an external antigen disturbing this network would be conditioned by the idiotypic interactions that already exist.

The concept of idiotypic networks has now been extended to incorporate helper and suppressor T cells. TCRs which recognize specific antigens may themselves contain idiotypes which in turn can be recognized either by antibodies or by other TCR-bearing T lymphocytes. The existence of such networks has provided a possible basis for manipulation of the immune response (Section 7.7.3).

4.4.4 Immunoglobulin heavy chain class-switching

During an immune response, antibodies can switch from one immunoglobulin-constant heavy-chain type to another. This is known as class switching and is largely under T cell control and mediated through the action of cytokines. *In vitro* cultures of splenic B lymphocytes stimulated with lipopolysaccharide (LPS) produce IgM, IgG3 and IgG2b immunoglobulins. The addition of IL-4 changes the response primarily to that of IgG1, mimicking the regulatory effects of T cells in establishing certain memory responses. Similarly, the addition of γ-interferon to LPS-stimulated B cells induces responses restricted to IgG2a. Expression of a heavy-chain isotype involves a deletion type recombination process which is distinct from V region assembly. This is mediated through a number of switch regions which are located at the 5' ends of each set of C region exons. Switch regions generally consist of short tandem sequence repeats.

4.4.5 Idiotypes and auto-antibodies

Auto-antibodies are a hallmark of autoimmune disease and often contribute to tissue damage. However, some auto-antibodies, such as those directed against DNA and IgG (rheumatoid factor, RF) are also often found in low concentrations in healthy people and may have a normal physiological function. Much information has come from investigating the idiotypic make-up of these auto-antibodies by the generation of anti-idiotypic antibodies. These have been used to facilitate the molecular characterization and cloning of the germline genes responsible for these idiotypes.

IgM myeloma and IgM paraproteins frequently have RF auto-antibody activity. Approximately 10% of patients with Waldenstrom's macroglobulinemia have IgM RF. This is remarkable considering the almost limitless potential of the B cell repertoire and that such malignancies are thought to be the result of chance clonal expansion of a lymphocyte population. An even more interesting discovery was that approximately 60% of IgM-RF paraproteins express the same idiotype, termed 'Wa'. Many more idiotypes have now been identified for both RFs and other auto-antibodies. Some corresponding V region genes have been identified and are summarized in *Table 4.1*. An idiotype designated 16/6 is present on a range of anti-DNA and other auto-antibodies. This idiotype has been detected with varying frequency in patients with a wide range of autoimmune, parasitic and infectious diseases.

The majority of RF idiotypes can be accounted for by a limited number of variable region genes, arguing against somatic mutation making a major contribution towards the generation of RF specificity. Considerable evidence now exists to indicate that RF-related V region immunoglobulin genes are rearranged and expressed early in the development of the immune system.

Table 4.1: *Human immunoglobulin variable region genes encoding auto-antibody idiotypes*

	V region	Auto-antibody
Heavy chain	VH783	Rheumatoid factor (RF)
	hv1051	RF, anti-cardiolipin
	VH4	RF
	hv3005	RF
	1.9111	Anti-DNA
	VH26	Anti-DNA, polyreactive
	9-1	Anti-Sm
	6-1G1	Polyreactive
Light chain	vg	RF, cold agglutinin, anti-DNA, anti-cardiolipin, RF, anti-DNA
	kv328h5	RF, anti-DNA
	iv117	RF, anti-DNA
	kv325	RF, cold agglutinin, anti-DNA, anti-intermediate filament, anti-low density lipoprotein

4.4.6 A possible physiological role for rheumatoid factor

There is evidence that auto-antibodies to IgG, DNA and bacterial polysaccharides are related in that they utilize the same or similar V region genes. RF can therefore be useful in amplifying immune responses to a range of micro-organisms. RF can bind strongly, and thus stabilize, IgG antibodies produced in an early polyclonal response, and which have low-affinity binding to bacterial antigens. This will promote activation of the complement pathway. IgM-RF is also important in the clearance of IgG immune complexes. This may be particularly relevant for IgG subclasses which do not fix complement.

Lymphocytes with RF cell surface receptors are abundant even in individuals with no or low levels of circulating RF. These RF precursor B cells are most frequent in the mantle zones of lymph nodes, regions where immune complexes often localize. It has been suggested that B cells expressing RF on their surface may have a role in processing and presenting antigens trapped in immune complexes.

A down side to this situation may occur if helper T cells, recognizing an epitope within the processed antigen, also provide a route for initiating a self-reactive process resulting in auto-antibody production. Repeated exposure to antigens which form immune complexes and contain a T cell epitope may provide the stimulus for the production of high titer RF.

4.4.7 Abnormal glycosylation of IgG

In recent years considerable interest has centered around variation in the N-glycosylation patterns of IgG and its possible involvement in autoimmunity. The carbohydrate moieties attached to the CH_2 domains of the IgG can be present in a shorter form ending in N-acetylglucosamine instead of galactose and sialic acid. The ratio of agalactosyl IgG to normal IgG increases with age and is also raised in RA, juvenile chronic arthritis and tuberculosis. Levels of agalactosyl IgG are also increased in animals with experimentally induced arthritis.

4.4.8 Hypergammaglobulinemia

The trigger for auto-antibody production is unclear. Current theories favor the concept that the production of auto-antibody is preceded by the development of auto-antigens. However, there is a school of thought which proposes that auto-antibodies are produced as a by-product of polyclonal B cell activation. In favor of this hypothesis is the fact that many autoimmune diseases are accompanied by polyclonal hypergammaglobulinemia. This is particularly true of Sjögren's Syndrome. This disease is associated with a selective polyclonal rise in IgG1. When one immunoglobulin class begins to rise at the expense of the others, especially if the others become subnormal, the clinician should be alerted to the possible development of malignancy (Section 7.2).

4.5 Methods of detecting auto-antibodies

A variety of methods can be used to detect the presence of auto-antibodies. Many are used routinely in clinical laboratories as an aid to diagnosis. Others are more specialized and have a more restricted use. Some tests are highly sensitive – that is, they detect the auto-antibody whenever it is present with no false negatives. Other tests are very specific – that is, they are only positive in one disease. Sensitivity is largely dependent on the assay used. Specificity depends on whether the auto-antibody concerned is produced in only one or in many conditions.

4.5.1 Immunofluorescence

Indirect immunofluorescence is used widely to identify organ-specific auto-anti-bodies (*Table 4.2*). The test is based on the histological identification of binding of auto-antibodies to a tissue section. The basic principle is summarized in *Figure 4.3*. Cryostat sections of various tissues are prepared to cover the range of auto-antibodies to be tested. Tissues regularly used include liver, thyroid, stomach, kidney, muscle and lip. These are prepared either from human autopsy samples or from sacrificed animals such as rats. Rather than have single slides for each tissue, composite slides of all tissues are sometimes made. Tissue sections are incubated with serum from the patient. Any organ-specific antibodies present will bind to the tissue. Following washing to remove the serum, the tissue section is incubated with an antibody raised in either sheep or rabbits against human immunoglobulin. The second antibody is conjugated to a fluorescent compound such as fluorescein isothiocyanate (FITC). This compound fluoresces bright apple green when exposed to ultraviolet radiation. After further washing, the tissue section is examined microscopically under ultraviolet radiation. Visible fluorescence signifies binding of auto-antibodies. The advantage of this technique is that the exact localization of the antibody–antigen complex can be seen, giving information about the identity of the auto-antigen. For example, the pattern of fluorescence in anti-nuclear antibody (ANA) tests can be homogeneous, speckled, nucleolar or perinuclear, depending on the auto-antigen recognized by the antibodies.

Variants of the indirect immunofluorescence test exist. One test now widely used detects ANAs by using HEP-2 cell lines. These cells are kept in continuous culture and, following trypsinization to remove them from culture flasks, are allowed to adhere to microscope slides. By using indirect immunofluorescence the different patterns of ANA staining can clearly be observed.

Direct immunofluorescence can be used on biopsy material to demonstrate whether auto-antibodies have already been deposited in the tissue *in vivo*. Cryostat sections of the biopsy are prepared, directly incubated with the FITC anti-human immunoglobulin and examined as before. This procedure is sometimes used to examine skin and kidney biopsies.

Table 4.2: *Auto-antibodies detected by immunofluorescence*

Tissue used	Auto-antibody detected	Associated diseases
Rat liver- hepatocytes	Anti-nuclear	SLE Sjögren's Syndrome, scleroderma, RA

Hep-2 cell line	Anti-nuclear	RA, SLE,
		  scleroderma,
		  Sjögren's Syndrome

Stomach	Anti-smooth muscle
	  (inter-gastric gland fibres)
		Chronic active
		  hepatitis

Stomach	Anti-parietal cells	Pernicious anemia

Stomach	Anti-reticulin
	  (inter-gastric gland interstitium)
		Celiac disease,
		  dermatitis
		  herpetiformis

Liver	Anti-mitochondrial
	  (cytoplasm of hepatocytes)
	Anti-microsomal
		Primary biliary
		  cirrhosis

Thyroid	Anti-thyroid peroxidase	Hashimoto's
		  thyroiditis,
		  Grave's Disease

Rat diaphragm	Skeletal muscle	?
Rat lip	Antibody to intercellular cement of stratified squamous epithelium	Pemphigus
Rat lip	Antibody to basement membrane of stratified squamous epithelium	Bullous pemphigoid
Human adrenal	Antibody to cytoplasm of cortical adrenal cells	Addison's Disease
Pancreas	Islet cell antibodies	Type I diabetes mellitus

4.5.2 Enzyme-linked immunosorbent assay (ELISA)

ELISA has become very popular over the last 10 years and has now largely superseded assays which use radioactive isotopes (*Table 4.3*). The main advantages of the ELISA technique are its sensitivity, the fact it can be quantitative, its ease and simplicity, its safety and the avoidance of radioactivity. The basic principle is summarized in *Figure 4.4*.

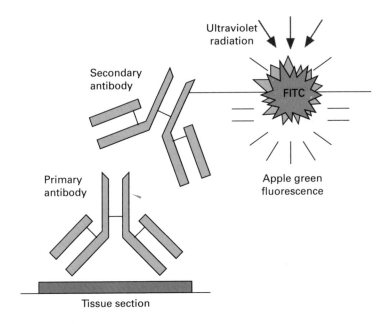

Figure 4.3: Indirect immunofluorescence.

   Wells of plastic microtiter plates are coated with the relevant antigen. This step has become more simple and reproducible as recombinant auto-antigens have become available. Synthetic peptides corresponding to major auto-antigenic epitopes can also be used to coat plates. Antigens will often bind spontaneously to the plastic plates. In other cases the plates can be pre-treated to 'induce' the antigen onto the plate. After the plates have been coated, they are incubated with an excess of non-specific protein such as bovine serum albumin, in order to saturate completely the plastic's ability to bind further protein.

   Dilutions of the patient's serum are made and fixed volumes are added to the antigen-coated wells. If auto-antibodies are present they will bind to the solid phase antigen. The plates are then washed to remove unbound antibodies and a second antibody added to each well. This is an anti-human-immunoglobulin which has been conjugated to an enzyme, usually horseradish peroxidase or alkaline phosphatase. Following this incubation the wells are washed again and an enzyme substrate is added. The presence of enzyme will change the substrate to produce a color reaction which can be measured quantitatively. Many sophisticated mechanized ELISA plate readers are now available which automatically read the color development and have in-built software to analyze the results. Known standards can be used to prepare a curve against which results can be calibrated. ELISA tests are very sensitive and it is important to have sufficient data on normal controls in order to decide where values exceed the normal range. Many auto-antibodies can be detected in this way, including antibodies to type II collagen and the extractable nuclear antigens Ro and La.

Table 4.3: *Auto-antibodies detected by either ELISA or radioisotopic assays*

Antibodies detected	Associated diseases
IgG,IgA,IgM rheumatoid factors	RA
Collagen (types I-IX)	RA (type II collagen)
Proteoglycan of cartilage	RA
Insulin	Type I diabetes mellitus
Acetylcholine receptor	Myasthenia gravis
Intrinsic factor	Pernicious anemia
Myeloperoxidase in primary granules of neutrophils (anti-neutrophil cytoplasmic antibodies)	Wegener's granulomatosis and systemic vasculitis
Enzyme components of mitochondria	Primary biliary cirrhosis
ds DNA	SLE
ENAs Ro La	SLE, Sjögrens Syndrome
Sm	SLE
Jo-1 Mi Pm-1	Polymyositis
Ku U1-RNP	Polymyositis/ scleroderma overlap

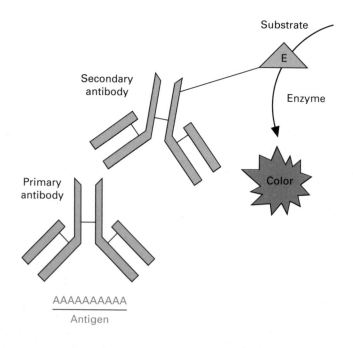

Figure 4.4: *ELISA.*

4.5.3 Passive agglutination

This method is based on the fact that antibodies can agglutinate and precipitate particles, such as latex or red blood cells, which have been coated with (auto)antigen. The test is usually performed in round or 'V' bottomed microtiter plates to which equal volumes of diluted patient's serum and the coated particle suspension are added. Negative and positive control sera must always be included in the assay.

Rheumatoid factors (anti-immunoglobulin) can be detected by their ability to agglutinate latex particles coated with human IgG. The sera from patients are tested at a range of dilutions with a positive test at 1/40 or 1/80 dilution being taken as clinically significant. IgM antibodies agglutinate best, although IgG antibodies can be detected to a lesser degree. Sheep red blood cells can also be coated with immunoglobulin and used to test for rheumatoid factor. This is known as the sheep red blood cell agglutination test or the Rose–Waaler Test.

Auto-antigens can be attached chemically to the surface of red blood cells. A variety of coating procedures can be used although the most popular involves chromic acid. Auto-antibodies to thyroid peroxidase and thyroglobulin can be detected by passive hemagglutination. Turkey red blood cells coated with these antigens are available commercially and can be used to screen both qualitatively and quantitatively for auto-antibodies to these antigens.

Agglutination of a patient's own red blood cells following a direct anti-globulin test is indicative of autoimmune hemolytic anemia. In patients with this condition the red cells are coated *in vivo* with anti-red cell antibodies. When Coomb's reagent (an anti-human immunoglobulin serum) is added to washed red cells taken from the patient, it cross-links the 'sensitized' cells and agglutination occurs signifying a positive result.

4.5.4 Radioisotopic methods

Although less favored, some tests still utilize radioactive isotopes to quantify auto-antibody levels. Assays may be based on direct binding of radiolabeled antigen or alternatively on indirect or competition assays.

Antibodies to double-stranded DNA can be measured in a direct binding assay. In this method DNA in *E. coli* is intrinsically labeled with a $[^{14}C]$DNA precursor. Radiolabeled DNA extract is incubated with diluted patient's serum. Any anti-DNA antibodies will bind to the antigen and the resulting immune complex can be precipitated in the globulin fraction by 50% saturated ammonium sulfate solution. The amount of binding can then be assessed by determining the level of radioactivity in the precipitate and expressing it as a percentage of the total label originally added to each sample.

Antibodies to intrinsic factor can be measured by an isotopic competition method. The principle of this assay is based on radioactive vitamin B12, which can subsequently be separated by absorption with activated charcoal. By comparing the counts in the charcoal deposit to those in the supernatant, the amount of antibody to intrinsic factor can be determined. Antibodies to intrinsic factor are only present in approximately two-thirds of pernicious anemia patients but they are highly specific for this disease.

4.5.5 Western blotting

Although Western blotting is rarely used routinely to identify auto-antibodies, it is a powerful technique for characterizing auto-antigens and auto-antibodies at a research level. The technique is based on separating extracts of auto-antigen by charge and size on polyacrylamide gels (*Figure 4.5*). This can be done with SDS detergent (reducing

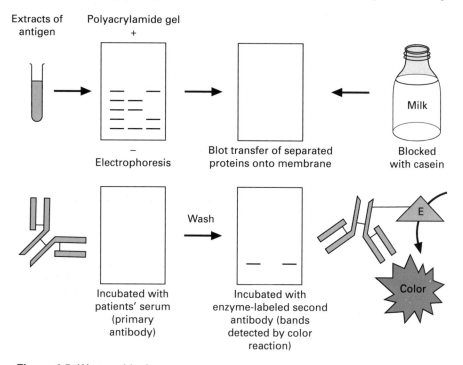

Figure 4.5: *Western blotting.*

conditions) or without (non-reducing). The addition of SDS will reduce any antigen with more than one chain into its individual components. Following separation, the resolved bands of antigen are transferred or blotted on to a solid membrane. This is usually nitrocellulose or nylon. The residual protein-binding ability of the membrane is blocked by incubation with bovine serum albumin or casein (dried milk powder). The membrane is incubated with the patient's serum or test sample with suspected antibody activity. Following washing, a second antibody (one which will react with the first), labeled with enzyme (usually horseradish peroxidase or alkaline phosphatase) is applied. On addition of the relevant substrate a color reaction will indicate which bands have reacted with the first antibody. Information regarding the molecular structure of the antigen can often be gained by comparing blots made under reducing and non-reducing conditions.

4.5.6 Assays using avidin–biotin

The interaction between biotin and avidin is one of the most useful modifications of immunochemistry which has been incorporated into ELISA, immunohistology and

Western blotting assays. An extremely high binding affinity exists between the water-soluble vitamin biotin and the egg-white protein avidin. This binding is undisturbed by extremes of pH buffer salts. The biotin molecule can easily be coupled to either antigens or antibodies, with complete retention of activity. Subsequently, avidin can be conjugated with enzymes or fluorochromes and used as a high-affinity secondary agent, which then greatly increases the sensitivity of an assay. Streptavidin, an extracellular protein of *Streptomyces avidinii*, is now often used in preference to avidin. This is because of its lower non-specific binding, largely due to its charge characteristics and low carbohydrate content (carbohydrates sometimes bind to lectins).

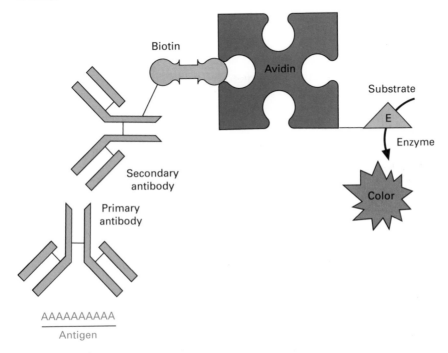

Figure 4.6: *Indirect labeled avidin–biotin assay.*

The most common use of avidin–biotin is in ELISA systems. Three basic assay designs are used:

- Labeled avidin-biotin (*Figure 4.6*). Antigen is bound to plastic plates and incubated with various concentrations of patient and control sera. Following washing, biotinylated secondary antibody is added. After incubation and washing the final stage is the addition of the avidin–enzyme complex. When substrate is added, the resulting color development correlates with the concentration of the primary antibody.

- Bridged avidin–biotin assay (*Figure 4.7*). This method is essentially the same but the avidin is not conjugated with enzyme. The avidin acts as a bridge between the biotinylated enzyme and the biotinylated secondary antibody. As avidin has multiple binding sites for biotin, more enzyme can be complexed, increasing the intensity of the substrate color development, making a more sensitive assay.

- Avidin–biotin complex assay (*Figure 4.8*). This variation requires the biotinylated enzyme to be pre-incubated with avidin, so that complexes of the two are formed. These can then be used as above with the complexes binding to biotinylated secondary antibody which has been immobilized to primary antibodies. This approach results in a greater concentration of enzyme on the surface of the well giving very sensitive assays.

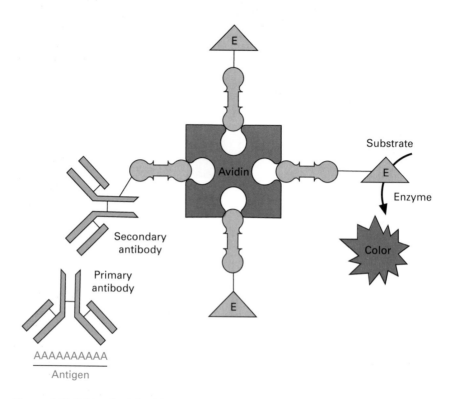

Figure 4.7: *Bridged avidin–biotin.*

4.5.7 Double immuno-diffusion and countercurrent immuno-electrophoresis

These techniques are routinely used in many laboratories to identify auto-antibodies, especially those directed to extractable nuclear antigens (ENAs). Double immuno-diffusion is a procedure where both antibody and antigen are allowed to migrate towards each other in an agarose gel. A line of precipitated immune complex forms where antibody and antigen reach equivalence. This position is determined by the relative concentrations of antibody and antigen and also by their molecular size (and thus the rate they will diffuse in the gel). A test gel is usually designed with a center well containing antigen surrounded by peripheral wells containing patients' sera and known antibody controls (*Figure 4.9*). Alternatively an antibody can be added to the center well with antigens in the peripheral wells. Such gels are often referred to as Ouchterlony plates.

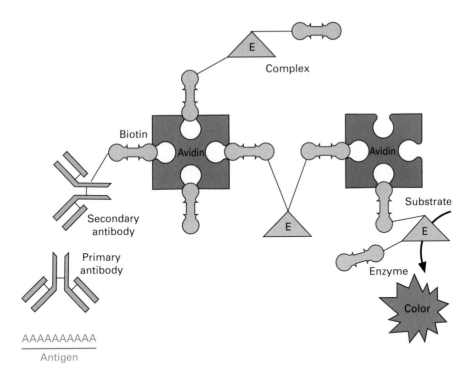

Figure 4.8: *Avidin–biotin complexes.*

In *Figure 4.9* a mixture of antigens has been used in the center well. If two sera (S_1, S_2) both contain the same antibody against an antigen and they are positioned adjacent to each other, the two lines of precipitation formed will merge smoothly. However, if adjacent sera (S_2, S_3) have antibodies recognizing different antigens, the two lines formed will cross each other. This can be used to characterize auto-antibodies to ENAs. A patient's serum with suspected auto-antibodies is put adjacent to wells containing control antibodies of known specificity (e.g. anti-Ro or anti-Sm) and tested against a crude extract of ENAs. By using a range of known controls it is possible to assign auto-antibody specificity.

Countercurrent immuno-electrophoresis, a more rapid and sensitive screening technique, is often used. This is similar to immuno-diffusion but by applying an electric current to the gel, the antibody and antigen can be driven towards each other, dramatically speeding up the test process (*Figure 4.10*). Immunoglobulins differ from most other proteins in that they migrate towards the cathode by electro-osmosis. This technique can therefore be used whenever the antigen is of a higher electrophoretic mobility than the antibody. Countercurrent immuno-electrophoresis can be used for detecting auto-antibodies to thyroglobulin and to ENAs.

For the detection of antibodies to ENAs, wells cut into the anodal side of the agar plate are filled with the patient's sera. A current is then applied for 10 or 15 minutes before the antigen extract is added to the cathodal wells or trough. This allows the relatively slow-moving antibodies to gain a 'head start' on the antigens. When the antigen extract is added to the cathodal wells the current is applied for a further 45

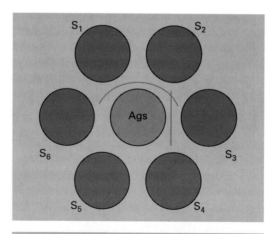

Lines of precipitated immune complexes are formed at a point of equivalence between antibodies and antigens. The line merges between S1 and S2 indicating they both contain an antibody recognizing the same antigen. The line between S2 and S3 crosses indicating they contain antibodies recognizing different antigens

Figure 4.9: Double immuno-diffusion – Ouchterlony plates.

minutes. Lines of precipitation are formed where the antigen–antibody molecules meet.

All ENAs cannot be prepared from a single tissue. Therefore sera are usually tested against extracts made from both human spleen and rabbit thymus. The ENA Scl-70 is found only in rabbit thymus extracts and not in human spleen preparations. The opposite is true for Ro (SSA) antigen. An extract of calf thymus is a good source of the Jo-1 antigen. For routine ENA screening, it is not usual to put control and test sera adjacent to each other and the controls are often randomly positioned. This is due to the relative scarcity of good control sera. When a precipitation is found between a patient's serum and the antigen extract, the test is usually run again with more extensive control sera, either in countercurrent immuno-electrophoresis or double immuno-diffusion.

4.6 The pathology of autoimmune diseases

There are three main immunopathologic processes involved in AD. In the first mechanism the auto-antibody is involved directly in the disease process. This is the underlying mechanism in autoimmune hemolytic anemia, Goodpasture's Syndrome and myasthenia gravis. Destruction of the cells or tissues concerned often ensues, generally through the binding of complement. The auto-antibody and complement can be demonstrated on the cells and tissues using direct immunofluorescence. The second mechanism is by the deposition of immune complexes. The size of these complexes is determined by the relative proportions of auto-antigen and auto-antibody. Immune complexes lodge, and can be demonstrated by immunofluorescence, in the microvasculature of a variety of organs (most commonly the skin, joints and kidneys)

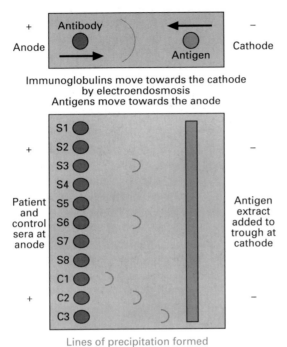

Figure 4.10: Countercurrent immuno-electrophoresis.

and provoke an inflammatory reaction. This type of pathology is common in SLE and in systemic rheumatoid arthritis. The third mechanism is direct organ damage by activated T lymphocytic infiltration followed by destruction, presumably mediated by lymphokines, of target cells. This is the predominant mechanism in most organ-specific ADs and in Sjögren's Syndrome.

Autoimmune processes become a 'disease' when pathological changes are detected. This may sometimes predate the observation of clinical signs. Characteristic pathology is largely determined by whether an organ specific or non-organ specific antigen is involved. Much of the pathology relating to specific conditions is detailed in Chapters 5 and 6.

Auto-antibodies can be involved in other damaging reactions through opsonization (antibody-induced phagocytosis) and ADCC. When auto-antibodies combine with cell surface antigen, their exposed Fc regions can combine with the Fc receptors of macrophages or lymphocytes. The former results in increased phagocytosis and the latter in ADCC. Both of these processes can contribute to overall tissue damage.

For pregnant women with AD an important concern is the possible passive transfer of auto-antibodies to the fetus. IgG auto-antibodies can cross the placenta. Sometimes the end-result is permanent (e.g. congenital heart block in babies of women with anti-Ro antibodies); in other situations the condition is transient (e.g. neonatal ITP).

Deposition of immune complexes can lead to a variety of pathological changes. These include inflammation of glomeruli in the kidney resulting in hypertension, in leakage of protein, and/or in renal failure. Deposition within blood vessel walls may produce vasculitis and gangrene of a variety of organs. When immune complexes are deposited they may also activate the complement pathway. Besides the accompanying tissue damage, complement by-products encourage an extensive infiltration with polymorphs and macrophages. Death of these cells leads to the release of lysosomal enzymes and destruction of the surrounding tissue, a process termed leukocytoclasis.

Organ-specific autoimmune pathology is typified by extensive infiltration with lymphocytes. The infiltrating cells are predominantly CD4-positive T cells although there are also CD8-positive T cells and to a lesser extent macrophages, polymorphs,

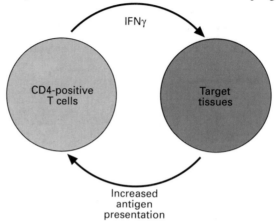

Figure 4.11: *Increased class II MHC expression.*

NK and plasma cells. The infiltration and its chronicity are driven by CD4-positive T cells which produce a variety of cytokines which in turn attract lymphocytes and macrophages into the area and promote their continued division and differentiation (Section 1.2.3). IFN-γ can act synergistically with TNF-α to up-regulate the expression of class II MHC molecules. Class II expression on tissues where it is not normally present is thought to be accompanied by an ability to present self-antigen and to add to the general immuno-inflammatory response. Thus once an autoimmune response is initiated release of cytokines may lead to a chain reaction (*Figure 4.11*). Although cytokines are usually produced and mediate their effect locally within the tissue, some may circulate and act on other tissues.

The precise mechanism of tissue destruction in organ-specific autoimmunity is not completely understood. However, it is thought that a number of different processes may be acting in concert. Given suitable cytokine signals, cytotoxic CD8-positive T cells can recognize auto-antigen in the context of self class I MHC molecules and destroy tissue cells. Cell-mediated cytotoxicity is thought to be a major cause of organ destruction in diseases such as Sjögren's Syndrome, thyroiditis and TI-DM.

Phospholipase A2 (PLA2) plays an important intracellular role in inflammatory processes and it is also now thought to be an extracellular mediator of inflammation. Soluble PLA2 has diverse biological roles in host defense, in amplification of inflammation and in the generation of lipid mediators. High levels of PLA2 activity have been found in the synovial fluid of rheumatoid arthritis patients.

Acute and chronic inflammation precipitated by autoimmunity and the presence of immune complexes can be initiated by the release of cytokines TNF, IL-1 and possibly IL-6 from a number of different cell types (predominantly macrophages). These cytokines induce a variety of cells, including osteoblasts, endothelial cells, synoviocytes and vascular smooth muscle cells, to synthesize and release PLA2. This in turn has a dramatic effect on a range of inflammatory mediators, such as lysosomal enzyme release, production of prostaglandins, increased production and release of lysophosphatides and reactive oxygen species. All of these can make a major contribution to the inflammatory processes taking place at a site of autoimmune destruction.

All of the processes described above may be involved in an individual AD to varying degrees. Many diseases are chronic with gradual destruction and loss of function of the target organ. This is usually accompanied by replacement of the tissue with fibrotic material.

Biopsies and histopathology can provide a wealth of information: whether the infiltration is predominantly lymphocytic or granulocytic; whether there is deposition of immune complexes; how much of the tissue has already been destroyed and fibrosed; and it can provide information on how active the disease process is at present.

4.7 Conclusion

Autoimmunity has both cellular and humoral components. The cellular aspects are mediated by cytotoxic T cells and NK cells. Both these cell types can lyse target cells. The humoral component of autoimmunity is the production of auto-antibodies by B cells. Most B cells require T cell help in order to produce auto-antibodies. CD5-positive B cells are an exception to this rule. There are various methods for detecting auto-antibodies in patients' sera. These include the use of immunofluorescence, ELISA techniques, radioisotopic methods and various types of immunodiffusion.

Within the human body three main immunopathologic processes can be identified. These are the direct involvement of auto-antibody; the deposition of immune complexes; and lymphocyte infiltration of specific organs.

Further reading

Hames, B.D. and Glover, D.M. (1988) *Molecular Immunology.* Frontiers in Molecular Biology. IRL Press, Oxford.

Hay, E.M., Freemont, A.J., Kay, R.A., Bernstein, R.M., Holt, P.J.L. and Pumphrey, R.S.H. (1990) Selective polyclonal increase of immunoglobulin G1 subclass: a link with Sjögren's Syndrome. *Ann. Rheum. Dis.,* **49**, 373.

Hecend, T. and Schmidt, R.E. (1988) Characteristics and uses of natural killer cells. *Immunol. Today,* **9**, 291.

Isenberg, D.A. and Maddison, P.J. (1987) Detection of antibodies to double stranded DNA and extractable nuclear antigen. *Broadsheet, Ass. Clin. Pathol.,* **117**, BMA Publications, London.

Isenberg, D.A. and Staines, N.A. (1990) DNA antibody idiotypes. An analysis of their role in health and disease. *J. Autoimmunity,* **3**, 339.

Johnstone, A. and Thorpe, R. (1987) *Immunochemistry in Practice.* Blackwell Scientific Publications, Oxford

Stoller, B.D. (1981) Anti-DNA antibodies, in *Clinics in Immunology and Allergy* (A.S. Fauci, ed.). W. B. Saunders and Co., London, pp. 243.

Thompson, R.A. (1981) *Techniques in Clinical Immunology.* Blackwell Scientific Publications, Oxford

Young, J.D.E. and Liu, C.C. (1988) Multiple mechanisms of lymphocyte mediated killing. *Immunol. Today,* **9**, 140.

5
CLINICAL CONSEQUENCES OF AUTOIMMUNITY: GENERAL CONSIDERATIONS AND MULTI-SYSTEM DISEASE

General considerations

5.1 Introduction

The first part of this book was concerned with current thinking about the causes and mechanisms underlying autoimmunity. The middle section of the book dealt with consequences of autoimmunity at a cellular and humoral level and also with the methods of measuring auto-antibodies. The next two chapters concern the manifestations of autoimmunity within the body – that is, with autoimmune diseases themselves. There are some diseases which quite clearly have an autoimmune basis (e.g. systemic lupus erythematosus, myxedema). In other diseases the role of autoimmunity is speculative. Our forebears tended to blame all diseases of unknown cause on evil humors or, later, on infections they had not yet identified. Our generation tends to attribute these same diseases to aberrations of the immune system. Thus inflammatory bowel disease, vasculitis and many other chronic diseases have been thought to have an autoimmune basis with little evidence as yet to support the theory. These two chapters are concerned predominantly with those conditions where there is clear evidence of autoimmunity.

Auto-antibodies can be divided into those which are organ specific (e.g. thyroid auto-antibodies) and those which are non-organ specific (e.g. anti-nuclear antibodies). The former tend to be associated with single organ diseases and the latter with multi-system disease. There are some areas of overlap – in Goodpasture's Syndrome, primary biliary cirrhosis and chronic active hepatitis non-organ specific antibodies are associated with diseases of relatively limited expression.

5.2 Epidemiology

Epidemiology is the study of the distribution and determinants of disease in specified populations. Epidemiologists seek to answer the following questions:

- how common is the disease?

- who gets it and why?

- what is the natural history of the disease?

Table 5.1: *Epidemiology of the autoimmune diseases*

Disease	Prevalence	Peak age at onset	Female:male	Racial variations
SLE	••	20–40	9 : 1	Commoner in Blacks and Chinese
Scleroderma	•	45–65	3 : 1	—
Polymyositis	•	45–65	2 : 1	—
RA	•••	35–50	3 : 1	Less in rural Blacks
Sjögren's Syndrome	••	50	9 : 1	—
Goodpasture's Syndrome	•	None	1 : 1	Commoner in Caucasians
Primary biliary cirrhosis	•	> 35	9 : 1	Rare in Africa, India, Middle East
Chronic active hepatitis	••	10–25, 50–60	3 : 1	—
Celiac disease	••	0.5-2; 50	1 : 1	Common W. Ireland
Pernicious anemia	•••	60–70	1.5 : 1	Common N. Europe
Autoimmune hemolytic anemia	•	> 50	1.5 : 1	—
ITP	•	20–40	4 : 1	—
Grave's Disease	•••	20–40	6 : 1	Commoner in developed countries
Hashimoto's thyroiditis	•••	40–60	9 : 1	—
Type 1 diabetes mellitus	•••	12–20	1 : 1	Common N.Europe, Rare in Asians
Pemphigus	•	40–60	1 : 1	Common Jews, Indians
Bullous pemphigoid	•	> 60	1 : 1	—
Dermatitis herpetiformis	•	20–40	1 : 1	—
Myasthenia gravis	•	20–30	3 : 1	—
Multiple sclerosis	•••	30	1.5 : 1	Increases with latitude

Prevalence key: • Rare <1 in 10,000, •• Uncommon <1 in 1000, ••• Common >1 in 1000

The study of disease frequency is important for the planning of health care provision. Differences in disease distribution between populations may provide clues to the etiology of the condition. For example, the frequency of multiple sclerosis increases with latitude (i.e. distance from the equator). This suggests that it may be caused by an environmental agent which is common in cold climates. Any theory about the causation of disease must take into account its observed epidemiology. Thus any theory of the cause of autoimmunity must be able to explain why most ADs are more common in women than men and why ADs appear to run in families. Differences in disease occurrence between populations may be due to genetic differences between the groups (the 'soil') or differences in exposure to certain environmental agents including infections (the 'seed') or a combination of both.

Disease frequency can be measured in a number of ways. The two methods referred to in this chapter are:

- disease incidence – the number of new cases of a condition during a given time period in a specified population;

- disease prevalence – the number of current cases of a condition at a particular time in a specified population.

Interesting features about the epidemiology of individual ADs will be discussed. *Table 5.1* summarizes the prevalence, peak age of onset, sex ratio and racial variation of the major conditions covered in these chapters. A quick glance will show that the

Table 5.2: *HLA associations with autoimmune conditions*

Disease	HLA alleles
SLE	DR3, DR2, B8, B5,
Scleroderma	DR5, B8
CREST syndrome	DR3
Polymyositis	B14, B8, DR3
RA	DR4(Dw4, Dw14) DR4(Dw15) (Orientals) DR1, DRw10 (Asians) DR9 (Chilean) B44, B15 B54 (Orientals)
Sjögren's Syndrome	A1, B8, DR3
Goodpasture's Syndrome	B7, DR2
Primary biliary cirrhosis	B8, DR3
Chronic active hepatitis	A1, B8, DR3
Celiac disease (and dermatitis herpetiformis)	A1, B8, DR3, DR7
Pernicious anemia	B7, B8, B18, Bw15 DR4, DR2, DR3
Autoimmune hemolytic anaemia	B8
ITP	DR2, B8, B12
Grave's Disease	B8, DR3 Bw46 (Chinese) Bw35 (Japanese)
Hashimoto's thyroiditis	B8, DR3
Type I diabetes mellitus	B8, B15, DR3, DR4 B54 (Orientals)
Pemphigus vulgaris	A26, B38, DR4(Dw10), DR6
Bullous pemphigoid	No known associations
Myasthenia gravis	A1, B8, DR3
Multiple sclerosis	A2, B7, DR2 (Dw2)

age of onset, sex ratio and prevalence of AD varies considerably, suggesting that each disease has a distinct set of etiological factors.

5.3 Genetics

Chapter 2 has covered the evidence for a genetic basis for autoimmunity. The specific genetic associations for the autoimmune diseases are summarized in *Table 5.2*. Some HLA associations recur (e.g. HLA A1, B8, DR3, DR4, DR2), others occur just once (e.g. DR5). Some ADs have been studied but only weak HLA associations have been found (e.g. primary biliary cirrhosis, pernicious anemia). An overview of this table, as of *Table 5.1*, shows that each AD must be considered separately. While it is possible to generalize about the genetic contribution to autoimmunity there is clearly no single gene defect which accounts for all ADs.

5.4 Overlap syndromes

Patients with a genetic predisposition to autoimmunity often develop more than one AD. In the case of the organ-specific AD it is clear that the patient has two conditions (e.g. hypothyroidism and pernicious anemia). These ADs tend to cluster in two distinct subgroups and these are described in more detail in Section 6.3.8. In the case of the multi-system ADs it is more difficult to say that the patient has two conditions (e.g. RA and SLE). What tends to happen is that they have features of both diseases producing a clinical picture which looks like neither disease. It can be argued that the multi-system ADs are not, in fact, a collection of different diseases but instead a single disease with a wide spectrum of manifestations. Certain manifestations frequently occur together and so are called distinct disease entities but patients may equally well straddle two of these so-called diseases. Such patients are said to have an 'overlap syndrome'. A schematic representation of the most commonly occurring overlaps is shown in *Figure 5.1*.

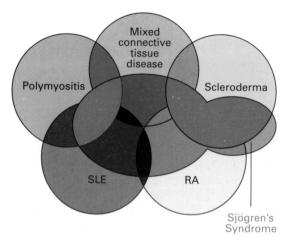

Figure 5.1: *Common overlaps in multi-system autoimmune diseases.*

Multi-system autoimmune disease

5.5 Systemic lupus erythematosus (SLE)

The word 'lupus' comes from the Latin word meaning wolf. The term has been used since medieval times to describe skin lesions which devour the flesh. In 1872 Kaposi distinguished two types of lupus erythematosus – a type confined to the skin and the multi-system type (SLE).

5.5.1 Immunology

The immunological hallmark of SLE is the presence of circulating ANAs (*Table 5.3*). These are present in 96% of cases. The ANA may be directed against various components of the nucleus, the most characteristic being native or double-stranded DNA (dsDNA). Anti-dsDNA antibodies are seldom found in any condition other than

Table 5.3: *Anti-nuclear antibodies found in SLE*

Antigen		Function	Frequency
dsDNA		Genetic material	60%
ssDNA		Genetic material	90%
Histones	H1, H2A, H2B H3, H4	Package DNA	70%
Sm	Proteins B, B1 D, E, F, G	RNA processing	4% in Caucasians 30% in Blacks and Chinese
RNP A,C	Proteins 68 kd	RNA processing	23%
Ku	p70 and p80 proteins and DNA	Transcriptional activation	10%
Ro	60-, 54-, 52-, 48 kd	RNA transport or translation control	35%
La	46 kd	Transport of RNA polymerase III transcripts	15%

SLE. Antibodies to single-stranded DNA are also found in SLE but are less specific. Anti-DNA antibodies give a homogeneous staining pattern in the fluorescent ANA test (Section 4.5.1). Antibodies to soluble portions of the nucleus may also be found in SLE. These may be detected using a nuclear saline extraction method and are known collectively as extractable nuclear antigens (ENAs). Subsequent analysis often shows these antigens to be made of a number of different proteins with a shared epitope. By a strange convention these antigens are often named from the first two letters of the surname of the patient in whom they were first discovered (e.g. Sm = Smith). Anti-Sm antibodies are highly specific for SLE.

The Ku antigen is a DNA–protein complex consisting of two proteins of approximately 70 and 80 kd (p70 and p80) that bind covalently to one another and to the end of dsDNA. p70 auto-antibodies are associated with Grave's Disease as well as with SLE. Anti-RNP antibodies react with a small ribonucleoprotein particle that contains U1-RNA. Anti-Sm antibodies recognize U1-RNA and particles containing U2-, U4-, U5- and U6-RNA. *In vitro* it appears that anti-Sm and anti-RNP antibodies can inhibit nuclear editing of RNA transcripts. However, there is no evidence that these auto-antibodies can penetrate cells *in vivo*.

Ro and La antibodies are strongly associated with the Sicca Syndrome in SLE and with Sjögren's Syndrome (Section 5.11). They are described in detail in the section on Sjögren's Syndrome. Anti-La antibodies in SLE are significantly associated with HLA-DR3, a later age of disease onset, a low frequency of kidney involvement and are invariably accompanied by anti-Ro. In contrast anti-RNP antibodies are associated with HLA-DR4. There are thus complex interactions between HLA antigens, auto-antibody production and clinical manifestations in SLE.

In addition to ANAs, auto-antibodies may also be found in SLE to other cells and cellular components (*Table 5.4*). Many patients have anti-phospholipid (anti-cardiolipin) antibodies. Phospholipids are important constituents of cell membrane, platelets and blood vessel walls. The Wassermann reaction test for syphilis uses a phospholipid as a substrate. As a result of their anti-cardiolipin antibodies many SLE patients have a false positive test for syphilis.

Table 5.4: *Other auto-antibodies associated with SLE*

Rheumatoid factor
Anti-red blood cells
Anti-platelets
Anti-neuronal cells
Anti-lymphocytes
Anti-phospholipid

In addition to this gamut of auto-antibodies SLE patients have evidence of defective T suppressor cell function. There is also abnormal delayed hypersensitivity on skin testing. There is a marked polyclonal B cell activation and an associated hypergammaglobulinemia. Complement is consumed during the formation of the immune complexes. Patients with active SLE usually have low complement levels. Some individuals with inherited complement deficiencies, notably C2, develop an SLE-like picture in the absence of DNA antibodies.

5.5.2 Immunopathology

SLE is one of the few ADs where it is possible to implicate auto-antibodies directly in the disease process. Immune complexes containing dsDNA and anti-dsDNA antibodies can be demonstrated in the circulation and lodged in the microvasculature of the skin, joint, kidney and lung. Immune complexes can be demonstrated by direct immunofluorescence of sun-exposed normal skin in 70% of SLE patients. Granular deposits of immunoglobulin and complement are seen at the dermo-epidermal junction. This is called the lupus band test.

5.5.3 Causes of SLE

Why do the nuclear components in the lupus patient become antigenic? In some patients drugs are to blame – most commonly hydralazine, isoniazid and procainamide. Many of these compounds have an aromatic amine group which is metabolized by acetylation. Similar compounds are found in hair dyes and some foodstuffs. In some animal models of SLE a C-type RNA virus is responsible for the disease. It is possible that a virus may also be responsible for human lupus but none has yet been identified.

It is also likely that ultraviolet radiation may denature DNA and render it antigenic. About 30% of SLE patients report an exacerbation of their symptoms by sunlight. Reactive oxygen species, which are released at sites of inflammation during the respiratory burst that accompanies phagocytosis, can also denature DNA.

While it seems most likely that the auto-antibodies are generated in response to an auto-antigen, a possible role for polyclonal activation cannot be discounted. It is still unclear why large macromolecular complexes (such as Sm) are frequent targets of auto-antibodies or why certain auto-antibodies are associated with particular manifestations of SLE.

5.5.4 Clinical manifestations of SLE (see **Figure 5.2**)

Skin and joints. The commonest features of SLE are inflammation of the skin (often in sun-exposed parts) and joints secondary to immune complex deposition. The arthritis of SLE is relatively mild and seldom damages the cartilage or causes deformities. The rash is often across the cheeks in a classical butterfly distribution. Occasionally the skin lesions are more severe and progress to ulcers or gangrene. Many patients develop diffuse or patchy hair loss.

The structure of the lining of the chest wall (pleura) and heart sac (pericardium) have some similarities to that of the joint lining (synovium). SLE patients may develop painful inflammation of these structures (pleurisy/pericarditis).

Kidney. The serious consequences of SLE arise mainly from involvement of the kidney, lung or brain. Various patterns of kidney damage may be caused by circulating immune complexes depending, in part, on their size. Two clinical syndromes may result from renal damage – one is kidney (renal) failure which may come on very suddenly, and the other is the nephrotic syndrome. In the latter situation the kidneys leak large amounts of albumin and the patient becomes edematous because there is no longer sufficient albumin in the circulation to maintain an adequate osmotic pressure. Kidney biopsy is required to assess the type of damage occurring.

Lung. Small blood vessel inflammation in the lungs may produce progressive breathlessness. The muscles of the chest wall and diaphragm may also become inflamed and weak.

Brain. Inflammation in the brain may produce fits, loss of consciousness or a variety of psychiatric syndromes. This is relatively uncommon.

Thrombosis. As a result of the anti-cardiolipin antibody which promotes coagulation, patients may develop recurrent thrombosis in the arteries or veins. These clots may cause strokes or heart attacks. In pregnant women small clots in the placenta may cause miscarriages.

Blood problems. Antibodies to red blood cells and platelets may be associated with anemia and bleeding, respectively.

As can be seen from this description the possible features of SLE are very diverse since any permutation of these features may occur together. In addition, patients may feel unwell with fever and weight loss. Sub-sets of disease may be associated with specific auto-antibody patterns.

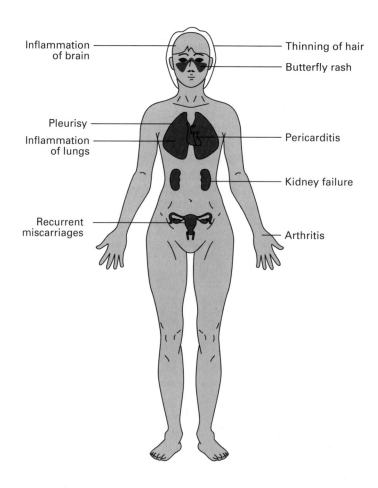

Figure 5.2: *Clinical features of SLE.*

5.5.5 Genetics

The most reproducible associations between SLE and HLA antigens have been demonstrated with A1, B5, B7, B8, DR2 and DR3. Further associations have been shown with null (silent) alleles of certain complement genes within the HLA class III region (C4A, C4B, C2). As reduced levels of complement components have been associated with a diminished ability to clear immune complexes, a biological rationale for these associations has been suggested. However, C4A*QO (the C4A null allele) is in strong linkage disequilibrium with DR3 and is found in the 'established' haplotype A1-Cw7-B8-DR3-C4A*QO-C4B*1-C2C-Bfs. This makes it difficult to assess the relative contributions of DR3 and C4A*QO towards susceptibility. Studies of SLE families have suggested that the major effect is due to class III region genes although this still has to be confirmed.

No association with DR3 is observed for SLE patients without anti-Ro and/or anti-La, suggesting that the HLA associations may be more with auto-antibody status than the disease *per se*. It has been suggested that the presence of these auto-antibodies correlates with combinations of DQA alleles possessing glutamine in position 34 of the first domain and DQB alleles having a leucine in position 26. Other studies have described an association between anti-Sm antibodies and DR2.

5.6 Scleroderma

Scleroderma means hardening and tightening of the skin. This may occur in a localized form or as part of a generalized condition called progressive systemic sclerosis (PSS) (*Table 5.5*).

Table 5.5: Classification of scleroderma

1. Generalized form with systemic involvement
   – progressive systemic sclerosis (PSS)
2. Limited form with little systemic change
   – CREST
3. Localized forms affecting small amounts of skin
   – morphea
   – linear scleroderma

5.6.1 Immunology

ANAs are found in approximately 75% of patients. The pattern under immunofluorescence is usually speckled or nucleolar. Twenty-three per cent of patients have anti-Scl 70 antibodies which are directed against DNA topoisomerase 1. This antibody is seldom found in any disease other than PSS. In contrast, CREST patients frequently have anti-centromere antibodies (95%) (see Section 5.7). Cultured lymphocytes from patients with PSS produce cytokines which are chemotactic for fibroblasts and enhance collagen production.

5.6.2 Immunopathology

PSS is associated with a progressive fibrosis due to the deposition of collagen in a variety of organs. In the initial phase an inflammatory response with lymphocytic infiltration is seen. Fibroblasts produce increased amounts of acid mucopolysaccharide which traps water and causes edema. Later the fibroblasts produce collagen. The epidermis becomes thinned and hair follicles and sweat glands are lost. The skin becomes thickened, shiny and tethered to the underlying tissues.

5.6.3 Causes of scleroderma

The cause of the excess collagen production is unknown but some accidents of nature provide interesting clues. Workers with vinyl chloride or silica may develop a scleroderma-like condition if they are genetically susceptible. An outbreak of scleroderma-like problems also occurred in Spain in 1981 and was attributed to

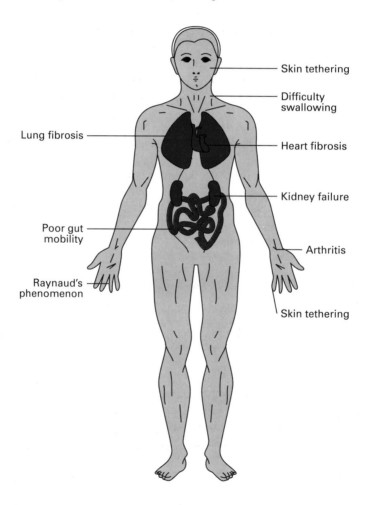

Figure 5.3: *Clinical features of scleroderma.*

adulterated cooking oil. A similar condition may also be seen in the recipients of bone marrow transplants (graft versus host disease). Some cases of scleroderma are drug induced (bleomycin, 5-hydroxytryptophan, pentazocine).

5.6.4 Clinical manifestations of PSS (see **Figure 5.3**)

One of the earliest features of PSS is the development of Raynaud's Phenomenon. This is a hypersensitivity of the fingers and toes to cold. The affected digit passes through a characteristic three-phase color change: first it goes white and looks dead, then it becomes blue and finally red as the blood flow returns. This condition may precede the onset of PSS by many years, gradually becoming more severe.

Skin. The skin changes begin in the fingers, toes and around the mouth and progress from there. As the condition worsens the fingers become fixed in a curled flexed position. Because of the poor blood supply the finger pulp diminishes and local infections and ulcers are common. Calcium deposits may occur in the skin which can be very painful. The skin has a characteristic waxy feel. Involvement of the skin around the mouth leads to difficulty in opening the mouth wide.

Joints. Joint pain and mild inflammation are common but severe arthritis is rare. The joints may become fixed partly due to the skin tethering and partly due to fibrosis within the joint.

Esophagus. Involvement of the esophagus is the commonest systemic involvement. Normal muscle activity is lost and it becomes difficult to swallow liquids in particular. Acid regurgitation from the stomach may also be a problem.

Gut. Diffuse fibrosis may occur throughout the gastrointestinal tract leading to reduced mobility. Bacteria may multiply in stagnant parts of the bowel using up vitamin supplies destined for the patient and causing malabsorption of food. Bloating, distension and constipation may ensue.

Lungs. Progressive fibrosis of the lungs may cause a dry cough and breathlessness. Occasionally cancers develop in the abnormal lung tissue.

Heart. Fibrosis of the heart may lead to rhythm disturbances and heart failure late in the disease.

Kidneys. Involvement of the small blood vessels of the kidney leads to high blood pressure as the body attempts to improve the perfusion of this vital organ. Uncontrollable high blood pressure was the most frequent cause of death in PSS before the advent of modern drug treatment. Often the only way to save the patient's life was to remove the kidneys and start dialysis. Renal failure still commonly occurs in PSS.

Nerves. Fibrosis may impinge on nerves causing local paralysis or numbness.

Muscles. Inflammation of muscles (myositis) frequently accompanies PSS.

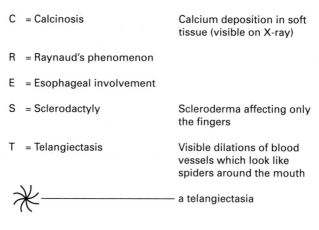

C = Calcinosis   Calcium deposition in soft
                                   tissue (visible on X-ray)

R = Raynaud's phenomenon

E = Esophageal involvement

S = Sclerodactyly   Scleroderma affecting only
                                   the fingers

T = Telangiectasis   Visible dilations of blood
                                   vessels which look like
                                   spiders around the mouth

                                   a telangiectasia

95% of patients with CREST have anti-centromere antibodies

Figure 5.4: *'CREST'.*

5.6.5 Genetics

Scleroderma is significantly but weakly associated with A9, B8 and DR5.

5.7 CREST

CREST is a benign variant of PSS. The acronym is explained in *Figure 5.4*. Although systemic involvement in this group of patients is very rare, occasionally the pulmonary arteries become fibrosed leading to right-sided heart failure.

5.8 Polymyositis/dermatomyositis

Autoimmune inflammatory disease of skeletal muscle may occur with associated skin involvement (dermatomyositis) or in isolation (polymyositis). In adults these conditions may be associated with an underlying tumor. Polymyositis may also occur in association with a number of other autoimmune diseases, particularly SLE, scleroderma and RA. Dermatomyositis is also a relatively common disease in childhood. Boys are slightly more commonly affected than girls.

5.8.1 Immunology

Auto-antibodies are commonly found in polymyositis (most commonly ANA). Four auto-antibodies have been described which are relatively specific for polymyositis. Two (Jo-1 and Mi) are found in polymyositis and two (PM-1 and Ku) in polymyositis–scleroderma overlap. Jo-1 is the most common of these (30% of patients), the antigen being histidyl-tRNA synthetase. Eighty per cent of patients with Jo-1 also have lung fibrosis and Raynaud's Phenomenon. Although many patients have these auto-antibodies it is unclear whether they play any causative part in the disease process.

Polymyositis seems to be mainly controlled by cell-mediated immunity. Peripheral blood lymphocytes from these patients are toxic *in vitro* to muscle cells. An association has been described between C2 deficiency (a component of complement) and polymyositis.

5.8.2 Immunopathology

In childhood dermatomyositis the primary lesion appears to be inflammation of small blood vessels supplying muscles. In adults the muscle tissue itself is inflamed with a marked B and T lymphocytic infiltrate. The muscle fibers show signs of degeneration and later of regeneration.

5.8.3 Causes of polymyositis

It is possible that a virus infection triggers the immunological reaction. Certain viruses are known to produce a similar illness, the most notable being the Coxsackie viruses. In about 8% of adult cases the disease is associated with cancer, usually of the lung, breast, ovary or stomach.

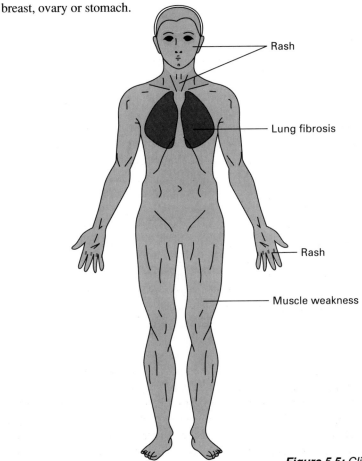

Figure 5.5: *Clinical features of dermatomyositis.*

5.8.4 Clinical manifestations: (see **Figure 5.5**)

The disease usually presents with weakness of the proximal muscles (those of the upper arm and upper leg). The speed of onset is quite variable. In about half the cases the muscles are also tender. If the weakness is widespread and severe the patient may have problems breathing or even die. The diagnosis can be confirmed by examining a muscle biopsy, looking at the electrical activity of the muscle (an electromyograph) or finding an elevated level of muscle enzymes in the blood. Two of these three tests must be positive to make a diagnosis. In the long term the diseased muscle may become heavily calcified. This is particularly common in childhood disease.

5.9 Mixed connective tissue disease

The term mixed connective tissue disease has been used to describe those patients with high levels of antibodies to nuclear ribonuclear protein (RNP). Anti-RNP antibodies are associated with HLA-DR4. These patients often have severe Raynaud's Phenomenon, arthritis, pleurisy, pericarditis and sclerodactyly. Pulmonary fibrosis and polymyositis are also common features. Whether this is indeed a separate disease entity or whether it represents an overlap syndrome between SLE and scleroderma is open to debate.

5.10 Rheumatoid arthritis

Although this condition is usually called RA it should, more correctly, be called rheumatoid disease because there are many systemic features. RA is a common disease affecting about 1 in 100 of the adult population. Overall, women are affected three times as often as men. The female to male ratio is higher in young adults than in those over 70 where the ratio is almost equal. RA may occur at any age but it is rare before puberty. The commonest age of onset is between 35 and 50. The disease frequency is fairly constant around the globe. There have been reports of reduced disease frequency in rural Black tribes.

5.10.1 Immunology

The characteristic auto-antibody of RA is rheumatoid factor (RF). RF is an antibody directed against the Fc portion of IgG. The most easily detected RFs (Section 4.5.3) belong to the IgM class. Eighty per cent of patients with RA have IgM RFs. The antibody is, however, not specific for RA and is found, usually in low titers, in many other connective tissue diseases and in chronic infections. Indeed RF production may play a role in normal immuno-regulation and homeostasis.

Many RA patients who do not have IgM RF (sero-negative patients) have RFs which belong to the IgG or IgA classes. Low titer ANAs are also common in RA. There is also evidence of defective cell-mediated immunity in this disease. Delayed skin hypersensitivity is abnormal and there is a functional deficit of T suppressor cells. This may, in turn, be related to abnormalities in the handling and production of interleukins.

The exact role which RF plays in the clinical manifestations of the disease is unclear. It is difficult to implicate RF in the destruction of cartilage and bone which is the most characteristic feature of RA.

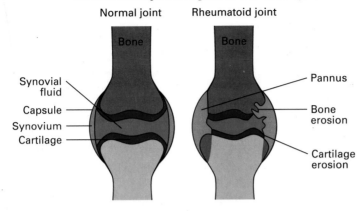

Figure 5.6: *Joints.*

5.10.2 Immunopathology

The synovium. RA is predominantly a disease of the lining of the joint – the synovium. Within 1 month of the onset of RA, the synovium shows thickening of the lining cell layer, vascular congestion and edema. As the disease progresses the sub-lining layer becomes densely infiltrated by lymphocytes, macrophages and plasma cells, often in nodular aggregates. These aggregates may have germinal centers so that the rheumatoid synovium has been likened to an ectopic lymph node.

Up to 85% of the infiltrating lymphocytes are T cells, although within the nodular aggregates B cells predominate. The synovium is rich in activated interdigitating macrophage-like cells which may be presenting antigen to CD4-positive T cells. These inducer cells may, in turn, permit B cell activation and immunoglobulin synthesis. There is clear evidence of both immunoglobulin and RF synthesis within the rheumatoid synovium. Lymphokines are also found within the joint cavity and these may stimulate collagenase release from synovial cells and augment the degradative process within the joint.

The thickened synovium is termed pannus (*Figure 5.6*). The protease and collagenase produced by the pannus erode cartilage and bone starting at the junction between cartilage and bone at the joint margin. These erosions can be seen on X-ray and progression of radiological erosions is one outcome measure used when assessing RA. Ultimately erosion of the bone and cartilage may lead to complete destruction of the joint.

Nodules. Patients with RA, especially those who are sero-positive, may develop nodules. These may occur anywhere in the body but are most common in the subcutaneous tissue over areas of pressure such as the elbow, the base of the spine and the Achilles tendon. Under the microscope they show a central necrotic area, surrounded by a palisade of mononuclear cells and with an outer capsule of chronic inflammatory cells.

5.10.3 Clinical manifestations

Joints. RA is characterized by inflammation of the synovial joints. It usually starts in the small joints of the hands (*Figure 5.7*) and feet. The most distal finger joints are

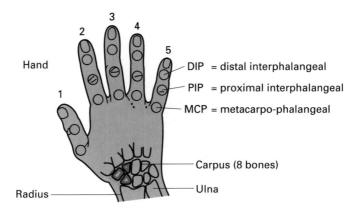

Figure 5.7: *Hand joints most commonly affected in early RA.*

usually spared. The joints of the second and third fingers are affected more commonly than the fourth and fifth. RA produces a symmetrical arthritis, meaning that the same joints are affected on both sides of the body. The larger joints such as the knee and elbow are affected later; and the hip may be spared for many years. The initial symptoms are joint pain, swelling and stiffness. These symptoms are usually at their worst in the early morning. Later the joints may become permanently deformed. The most typical deformity is ulnar deviation of the fingers (sideways displacement towards the ulna). The deformities often result in progressive disability.

Extra-articular features. Many patients with RA have disease confined to the joints. Even in these patients chronic tiredness, weight loss and mild fever may be a problem. Other patients may have evidence of the rheumatoid process outside the joints (*Figure 5.8*). The commonest extra-articular features of RA are nodules and enlarged lymph nodes. Nodules will occur at some stage of the disease in 25% of patients. Inflammation of the pleura (lung lining) and pericardium (heart sac) are also quite common. The inflammation may be associated with the production of fluid with a high fibrin content. Adhesions may form between the heart sac and the heart causing constrictive pericarditis.

Many patients with RA have associated Sjögren's Syndrome (Section 5.11) with dry eyes and a dry mouth. In addition they may develop inflammation of the white of the eye (scleritis). As a result of the inflammation this layer may become thinned (scleromalacia) or may even perforate, causing blindness (scleromalacia perforans).

As a result of circulating immune complexes lodging in the blood vessels patients with RA may develop vasculitis. Rheumatoid vasculitis may affect any organ but occurs most commonly in the small blood vessels of the skin causing gangrene of the fingers or toes or punched-out looking ulcers. One of the most serious extra-articular complications of RA is Felty's Syndrome. This affects about 0.5% of RA patients. Patients with Felty's Syndrome have enlarged spleens and low white cell counts (neutropenia). Their RA is usually very severe. The neutropenia renders them highly susceptible to infection.

Long term complications. Joint destruction and disability have already been mentioned. Any patient with a chronic inflammatory condition such as RA is susceptible

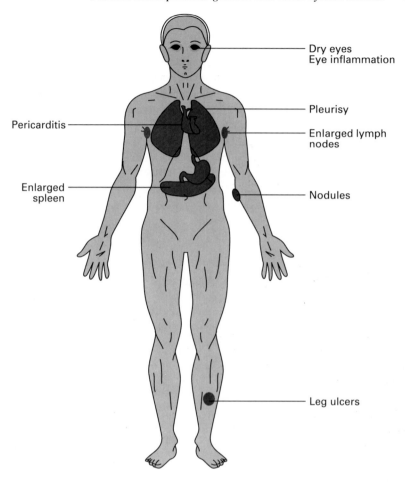

Dry eyes
Eye inflammation

Pleurisy

Pericarditis

Enlarged lymph
nodes

Enlarged
spleen

Nodules

Leg ulcers

Figure 5.8: *The extra-articular features of RA.*

to the development of amyloidosis. In this condition serum amyloid A protein (part of the acute phase response) is deposited in many organs including the kidney and may cause death as a result of kidney failure.

5.10.4 Genetics

RA is associated with Dw4 and DR4. In most studies a DR4 frequency of around 60–70% is found in RA patients, compared with 25% in controls. However, it is still unclear whether DR4 is a marker for disease susceptibility or severity in RA. Higher frequencies of DR4 are observed in RA patients with severe arthritis and in those developing extra-articular manifestations such as vasculitis and Felty's Syndrome. In Felty's Syndrome a frequency of almost 100% DR4 has been reported. Most studies have been in hospital patients. In contrast, at the population level no obvious association between RA and DR4 is seen, although the antigen frequency is raised in patients with erosive disease.

Whilst RA is associated with DR4 in many populations, several interesting exceptions have been found. RA is associated with DR1 in Israeli Jews and with DR9 in Chileans. Both DR1 and DRw10 are associated with RA in Asian Indian patients. In the Japanese, although RA is associated with DR4, it is with a particular subtype – Dw15. (On the basis of DRβ_1 amino acid sequences, DR4 can be sub-divided into Dw4, Dw10, Dw13, Dw14 and Dw15. More recently even more variants have been described.) In most caucasoid populations the DR4 variants associated with RA are Dw4 and Dw14. Dw10 never appears to be associated with RA, even in Jewish populations where Dw10 is the most frequent DR4 subtype. These observations have led to the formulation of a unifying hypothesis. The DRβ_1 chains of DR1, DR9, DRw10 and the DR4 variants Dw4, Dw14 and Dw15 all have a very similar sequence of basic amino acid residues in the third hypervariable region of the molecule (a shared epitope) (*Table 5.6*). This region is thought to be critical in determining how the peptide fits inside the α-helices of the DR molecule and consequently how it is presented to the T cell receptor (*Figure 5.9*).

Table 5.6: The association of HLA with RA appears to be with a shared epitope in the DRB third hypervariable region

		65	70
RA associated	DR4/Dw4	K D L L E Q K R A A	
	DR4/Dw14	K D L L E Q R R A A	
	DR4/Dw15	K D L L E Q R R A A	
	DR1/Dw1	K D L L E Q R R A A	
	DR9	K D L L E Q K R A A	
	DRw10	K D L L E R R R A A	
Non-associated	DR/Dw10	I D L L E D E R A A	

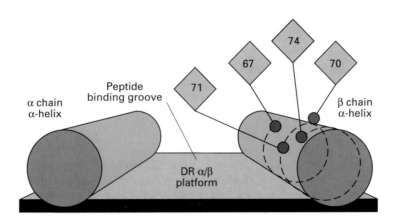

Figure 5.9: Peptide binding groove in the DR molecule.

5.11 Sjögren's Syndrome

Sjögren's Syndrome (SS) is a chronic AD affecting predominantly the exocrine glands. The glands are infiltrated with lymphocytes and plasma cells leading to diminished function. The tear and salivary glands are most commonly affected producing the characteristic symptoms first described by Henrich Sjögren in 1933: dry eyes (keratoconjunctivitis sicca) and dry mouth (xerostomia). SS may either occur on its own (in which case it is called primary SS) or in association with another AD (in which case it is called secondary SS). The most commonly associated ADs are RA and SLE.

The prevalence of primary SS in the general population is unknown. SS occurs in approximately 15% of RA patients, 40% of SLE patients, 70% of patients with primary biliary cirrhosis (Section 6.1.1) and 35% of patients with chronic active hepatitis (Section 6.1.2). SS may affect all ages, including children.

5.11.1 Immunology

Patients with SS usually have multiple auto-antibodies. RFs of the IgG, IgA and IgM classes have all been demonstrated in serum and saliva of patients with primary SS. Over 50% of patients also have marked hypergammaglobulinemia. Usually the immunoglobulins are polyclonal but monoclonal IgM may be seen. A fall in the level of IgM may herald the development of a malignancy (Section 7.2).

Eighty-five per cent of patients with primary SS have anti-Ro antibodies and 60% have anti-La antibodies. Both of these are ENAs. Much work has been done in recent years on the structure of the Ro and La antigens. Ro is an RNA–protein particle. The antigenicity is carried by a 60 kd protein bound to RNAs. Anti-Ro is almost invariably present in sera positive for anti-La, but may also occur alone. Transplacental passage of anti-Ro can produce heart block in the fetus. Anti-Ro antibodies are associated with the HLA genes DR2, DQ1 and DR3.

The La antigen is a peptide of 46–48 kd. A structural model has been constructed that shows La as a two-domain ribonucleoprotein with a larger domain of 28–29 kd bound to the tail of a small RNA. La is involved in transcription termination by RNA polymerase III. Up to 90% of patients with anti-La are DR3-positive. Anti-Ro and anti-La are common in primary SS but very rare in SS occurring in association with RA.

As in the case of SLE there is debate in SS as to whether the auto-antibody production occurs as a result of polyclonal activation or is antigen-driven. Patients with SS have been shown to have depressed T and natural killer cell function, as well as B cell hyperactivity.

5.11.2 Immunopathology

The affected glands show focal infiltrates of mononuclear cells. The glands become enlarged. The majority of lymphocytes are of the CD4 subtype with relatively few CD8-positive cells. Many of these cells show class II expression. Some may be CD4-positive cytotoxic T cells and directly involved in the destruction of the epithelium of the gland. Clonally expanded salivary gland lymphocytes have been detected in SS patients who later developed non-Hodgkin's lymphoma (Section 7.2).

5.11.3 Clinical manifestations

Glandular symptoms. In most patients lymphoproliferation is confined to the tear and salivary glands. They complain of eye discomfort (sandiness/grittiness). The tears are defective in quality as well as quantity. Lack of adequate lubrication of the eyes leads to an increased risk of abrasion and inability to wear contact lenses. Lack of saliva leads to difficulty in chewing, swallowing and speaking. Patients often have severe dental decay. A dry mouth can be detected by the 'cream cracker' test, an inability to eat this dry food without fluid. About half the patients with xerostomia exhibit intermittent swelling of the parotid glands giving them a 'chipmunk' appearance. Standard ways of quantifying tear and saliva production exist. To make a diagnosis of SS patients must have both keratoconjunctivitis sicca and xerostomia.

Extra-glandular symptoms. Occasionally, the lymphoproliferation of SS may affect exocrine glands in the respiratory tract, vagina, pancreas and bladder. Inadequate lubrication of these organs may produce symptoms. In addition, patients with primary SS may occasionally have features which are not attributable to the exocrine glands. The most common of these is a chronic arthritis which unlike RA, does not erode the cartilage or bone. Problems within the central nervous system and the kidney are the next most frequent features. The central nervous symptoms described include migraine, psychiatric abnormalities and malfunction of peripheral nerves. About one-fifth of patients with primary SS have renal tubular acidosis. This is an inability to acidify the urine causing retention of hydrogen ions (metabolic acidosis). As a result less calcium is bound to protein and calcium filtration is increased. This in turn may lead to kidney stones. Finally, patients with primary SS may develop lung inflammation and fibrosis. The lymphoma which complicates SS may sometimes originate from the lung.

5.11.4 Genetics

An association exists between DR3 and SS although, as with SLE, the underlying association appears to be predominantly with the presence of anti-Ro and anti-La antibodies. The highest levels of antibodies tend to be found in DQw1/DQw2 heterozygote patients. An association with DRw52 has been in anti-Ro/La-negative patients. No association with DP alleles has as yet been found.

5.12 Goodpasture's Syndrome

Goodpasture's Syndrome is characterized by rapidly progressive glomerulonephritis (inflammation of the kidney) and lung hemorrhage. The disease accounts for 2% of all cases of glomerulonephritis and can affect all ages and both sexes. It occurs mainly in Caucasians. The disease may follow acute respiratory infections or exposure to hydrocarbons. These agents may damage the basement membrane of cells within the lungs rendering them antigenic.

5.12.1 Immunology

The disease is characterized by high levels of circulating anti-basement membrane antibodies which are directly implicated in the disease process. Rapid removal of these antibodies by plasma exchange may lead to recovery in what is often a fatal disease. The anti-basement membrane antibodies react with epitopes which are common to the alveolar (lung) and glomerular (kidney) basement membrane. The antibodies are deposited in a smooth linear fashion.

5.12.2 Clinical manifestations

Patients usually present with rapidly progressive renal failure. They may also have loin pain and blood in the urine. About two-thirds of patients (usually smokers) also develop lung hemorrhage. This may be severe and life-threatening. Symptoms outside the lung or kidneys are rare.

5.13 Conclusions

There are a large number of ADs. This chapter has looked at those ADs which are non-organ specific. These conditions have in common a wide range of auto-antibodies most of which are directed against cellular components. The majority of the conditions affect multiple organs and may shorten life.

Further reading

Chapel, H. and Haeney, M. (1984) *Essentials of Clinical Immunology.* Blackwell Scientific Publications, Oxford.

Polednak, A.P. (1989) *Racial and Ethnic Differences of Disease.* Oxford University Press, Oxford.

Rose, N. and Machay, I (1985) *Autoimmune Diseases.* Academic Press, New York.

Schoenfeld, Y. and Isenberg, D. (1989) *The Mosaic of Autoimmunity.* Elsevier, Amsterdam.

Stiles, D.P., Stobo, J.D., Fudenberg, H.H., Wells, J.V. and Lange (1990) *Basic and Clinical Immunology.* Appleton and Lange.

Tiwari, J.L. and Terasaki, P.I. (1985) *HLA and Disease Associations.* Springer-Verlag, New York.

Weatherall, D.J., Ledingham, J.G.G. and Warrell, D.A. (1987) *Oxford Textbook of Medicine*, 2nd edn. Oxford University Press, Oxford.

6

CLINICAL CONSEQUENCES OF AUTOIMMUNITY: AUTOIMMUNE DISEASE OF PREDOMINANTLY ONE ORGAN

6.1 Gastrointestinal system

6.1.1 Primary biliary cirrhosis

Primary biliary cirrhosis (PBC) is an AD of the bile ducts within the substance of the liver. These ducts are progressively destroyed. There is a weak association with DR3.

Immunology. Almost 100% of patients with PBC have circulating auto-antibodies to constituents of mitochondria. The auto-antigens are non-organ and non-species specific. They are situated on the inner mitochondrial membrane. One antigen which seems to be specific for PBC is termed M2. M2 is part of the pyruvate dehydrogenase complex. Four polypeptide components of this complex have been identified. They are:

- E1 – 50 kd 2-oxyacid dehydrogenase complex

- E2 – 74 kd complex of lipoamide acyltransferase

- E3 – 50 kd 2-oxoglutarate complex

- Protein X – 52 kd (cross-reacts with E2)

  Ninety-four per cent of patients with PBC have antibodies either to E2 or to protein X. E2 is highly conserved in evolution, being present in the cells of bacteria through to mammals. Anti-mitochondrial antibodies (AMA) from PBC patients cross-react with subcellular constituents of bacteria including *E. coli*, *Klebsiella pneumoniae* and *Proteus sp*. E3 is found on the membrane of some archaebacteria and eubacteria. It is thus possible that antibodies to these structures, perhaps following intestinal infection, may cross-react with structures on bile duct epithelium. There have been reports of increased levels of rough (R) forms of *E. coli* in the stools of patients with PBC. AMA in low titer may also rarely be found in other ADs. Patients with PBC may also have high levels of ANAs and thyroid auto-antibodies. PBC is also associated with depressed T cell function.

Immunopathology. The earliest lesion of PBC is inflammatory destruction of the bile ducts within the liver. There is a heavy infiltrate of lymphocytes and plasma cells. Later granulomata develop and the bile ducts become fibrosed, and then cirrhosis may become established.

Clinical features. The disease may have a long symptom-free phase, having been diagnosed incidentally from abnormal blood tests. The earliest symptom is often intense itching which is attributed to retained bile salts in the circulation. Later the patient may become jaundiced. The level of cholesterol in the blood is markedly elevated and cholesterol may deposit in nodules in the skin especially around the eyes. Absence of bile salts within the bowel may lead to malabsorption of fatty foods and of the fat-soluble vitamin, vitamin D. This in turn may lead to thinning of the bones (osteomalacia) and bone pain. Liver failure ultimately occurs, often after 10–15 years. No drug therapy has been shown to improve survival in PBC. Once liver failure has occurred, liver transplantation is the only procedure that will save the patient's life. PBC is the most common indication for liver transplantation in Europe and accounts for 40% of such operations. The disease seldom recurs post-transplantation.

Associated diseases. PBC is frequently associated with other ADs; notably RA, scleroderma, CREST and autoimmune thyroiditis. Over 70% of patients with PBC have Sjögren's Syndrome.

6.1.2 Chronic active hepatitis (CAH)

Chronic hepatitis is defined as inflammation of the liver cells lasting for more than 6 months. There are many causes of chronic hepatitis: persistent viral infection (especially with hepatitis B), drugs, alcohol and an inability to handle copper ions. When all other causes have been excluded there remains a group of patients whose chronic hepatitis appears to have an autoimmune basis. This so-called CAH is probably due to a defective immunoregulatory system allowing an exaggerated response to a liver membrane antigen.

Immunology. Patients with CAH usually have high titers of ANAs (at one time the disease was called lupoid hepatitis) and auto-antibodies directed against smooth muscle (SMAs), liver cell membrane antigens or liver-specific proteins (LSPs). Hypergammaglobulinemia is a common finding.

The ANAs in CAH are directed against lamins: major nuclear proteins which form a filamentous network coating the inner surface of the nuclear envelope. Thus in the immunofluorescent ANA test these antibodies give a ring-like staining pattern around the periphery of the nucleus. LSP is an antigenic lipoprotein complex located on the plasma membrane of liver cells. The SMAs in CAH are directed against actin. CAH can be divided into two types: those with SMA (Type I – about 60%) and those without (Type II). The latter group are usually children or young adults. They have auto-antibodies directed against liver and kidney microsomes (LKMs). At least three LKM antibodies have been recognized. Recently part of the measles virus genome has been found to persist in the lymphocytes of patients with CAH suggesting that measles may play a role in the etiology of the disease.

Immunopathology. The liver is enlarged in the early stages. Later it shrinks and becomes cirrhotic. The liver cells are initially swollen and there is infiltration with plasma cells and lymphocytes. Fibrosis occurs after that, which tends to divide the liver into nodules. The liver cells then degenerate in a patchy fashion.

Clinical features. The disease has an insidious onset with several months of general malaise before jaundice is first noticed. The liver is usually normal in size by this stage but the spleen may be enlarged. In women the menstrual periods almost always cease. Approximately half the patients have symptoms from outside the liver – joint pains, skin rashes, bowel inflammation and shortness of breath. Untreated the condition has a chronic course with relapses and remissions leading to death from liver failure after 4–5 years. However, many patients respond well to immunosuppressive therapy.

Associated diseases. Many patients (60%) have other ADs especially autoimmune thyroiditis, diabetes and hemolytic anemia. Approximately 35% of patients with CAH have secondary SS.

6.1.3 Celiac disease

Celiac disease, an immunologically mediated condition of the intestinal mucosa, is triggered in genetically susceptible people by gluten. Gluten is a protein found in various forms of grain including wheat, barley and rye. The toxic fraction of gluten is α-gliadin. It is debatable whether celiac disease is truly an 'auto'-immune disease.

Epidemiology. There are two peak ages of onset of celiac disease. The first is in early childhood (aged 6–24 months) and the second is in middle age. The disease is particularly common on the west coast of Ireland. Over recent years there has been a trend towards later presentation in children.

Immunology. Many patients have α-gliadin antibodies in their circulation. These are not, however, specific for celiac disease. More specific are IgA endomysial antibodies. In addition many patients (60%) have anti-reticulin antibodies.

Immunopathology. The normal lining of the upper small intestine (jejunum) is composed of finger-like projections (villi) which are several times as long as they are wide. In celiac disease these villi are lost – a condition described as subvillous atrophy – and the lining is flat. There is an increase in IgM plasma cells.

Clinical features. The most common presenting features are diarrhea and malnutrition. The stools are bulky with a high fat content (steatorrhea). Many essential nutrients and vitamins are not absorbed and the patient loses weight and becomes anemic.

Associated diseases. Thyroid disease, TI-DM and other ADs occur with increased frequency in patients with celiac disease.

Genetics. HLA antigen associations have been found between celiac disease and DR3, DR7. These associations may be due to underlying linkage disequilibrium with DQw2. This specificity is associated with DR3 and a proportion of DR7 haplotypes. The majority of DR7 celiac patients (and all of the DR3 ones) are DQw2-positive, having the DQB2 allele at the DQβ locus. Further studies have demonstrated celiac disease to be associated with the DQA allele, DQA4, which is common to DR3, DR5 and DR8 haplotypes.

The DQA4/DQB2 heterodimer (the DQ surface molecule is made up of both α and β chains) will be encoded *in cis* on DR3 haplotypes and *in trans* in DR5/DR7 and DR8/DR7 genotypes. Observations so far are consistent with this DQA4/DQB2 heterodimer being an important risk factor for celiac disease.

More recent studies have implicated alleles of the DPB locus, namely DPB4.2 and DPB3, in celiac disease susceptibility. Comparison of DPB sequences suggests that amino acids at positions 56, 57 and 69 may be critical residues. The association of these DPB alleles appears to be completely independent of DR and DQ alleles, suggesting that there may be more than one susceptibility gene encoded with HLA.

It has been shown that these gene products do not bind α-gliadin nor are there any shared antigenic determinants between them. However, there is a degree of homology between an 8-amino acid sequence in α-gliadin and a 12-amino acid sequence in the 58 kd protein encoded in the region E1B of adenovirus 12. Thus a virus may also be involved in the pathogenesis of celiac disease.

Treatment. Celiac disease must be treated by a gluten-free diet. This is essential even in mild cases because celiac disease is associated with an increased risk of intestinal lymphoma. It has been shown that a gluten-free diet reduces this risk.

6.2 Hemopoietic system

6.2.1 Pernicious anemia

Pernicious anemia (PA) might, in fact, have been considered as an AD of the gastrointestinal tract. The anemia is due to a deficiency of vitamin B12. In normal circumstances the parietal cells of the stomach produce both hydrochloric acid and a carrier glycoprotein called intrinsic factor. Vitamin B12, a cobalt-containing vitamin, binds to intrinsic factor in the stomach and they travel together to the terminal ileum where the complex attaches to a specific receptor. Within the ileal cell B12 separates from intrinsic factor and binds to another carrier protein called transcobalamin II. This complex then enters the blood stream. B12 is a co-enzyme in the synthesis of methionine and succinic acid. It is also involved in the control of folate metabolism. A deficiency of B12 leads to a megaloblastic anemia and abnormal functioning of the nervous system. In PA the B12 deficiency results from the action of auto-antibodies to intrinsic factor and gastric parietal cells.

Epidemiology. Pernicious anemia is a common AD. The overall prevalence in Northern Europe is 1–2 per 1000. It is predominantly a disease of old age with very few cases occurring in those aged under 40, and a peak incidence in the 60s. Thus the prevalence in those aged over 70 is 3%. Even within the U.K. there are regional differences. The disease is three times as common in Scotland as in South-East England. It occurs in all races but is most common in northern Europeans, especially those with white hair and blue eyes. Women are affected slightly more commonly than men. There is a weak association with DR2, DR3, and DR4. However, over one-third of patients have a family history of PA or autoimmune thyroid disease. Many patients with PA have overt autoimmune thyroid disease and 55% have thyroid auto-antibodies.

Immunology. Antibodies to gastric parietal cells (GPCs) are found in 90% of patients with PA and can be demonstrated by immunofluorescence (Section 4.5.1). In addition, 50% of patients have antibodies directed against intrinsic factor (IF). There are two types of IF antibodies. Type I (blocking antibodies) are directed against the B12 binding site on IF and Type II are directed against the binding site for IF in the ileum. Type II IF antibodies are found in 35% of patients with PA (but only in those who also have Type I antibodies). IF antibodies are specific for PA whereas GPC antibodies are found in many diseases, especially Hashimoto's thyroiditis.

Immunopathology. The changes in the stomach are confined to the body and fundus (*Figure 6.1*). The walls are infiltrated with plasma cells and lymphocytes (predominantly CD8-positive cells). The other cells of the stomach wall become atrophied.

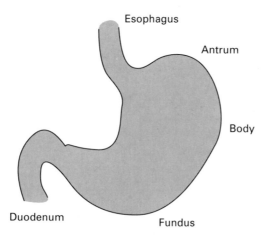

Figure 6.1: *Representation of the stomach.*

Clinical features. Intrinsic factor production has to be 1% of normal before B12 absorption is significantly affected. Thus PA has a very insidious onset. The usual presenting features are those of anemia (fatigue, breathlessness, weakness). The patient may be mildly jaundiced. In some cases a visual disturbance or psychiatric features may develop. Cancer of the stomach occurs in about 4% of cases (a threefold increased risk compared with the general population). Due to malfunctioning of the peripheral nerves patients may complain of tingling in the hands and feet; or difficulty in walking.

Treatment. PA responds to injections of vitamin B12. These need only be given once a month as vitamin B12 can be stored in the liver.

6.2.2 Autoimmune hemolytic anemia (AIHA)

Hemolysis is defined as the reduction of the average life span of the red blood cell below 120 days. A healthy bone marrow can compensate for mild degrees of hemolysis by increased cell production. However, once the life span of the red cell falls below a critical level (15 days for a healthy marrow) anemia is inevitable. Hemolysis may occur either because of an abnormality in the structure or function of the red cells, or because of increased destruction of normal red cells (usually by an over-active spleen). AIHA occurs because the red cells become coated with anti-red cell antibodies. The auto-antibodies can be divided into those which are most active at body temperature (37°C) (warm antibodies) and those which are most active at low temperatures (cold antibodies). Warm antibodies account for approximately 75% of red cell auto-antibodies. AIHA may occur either alone or as part of another disease (*Table 6.1*).

Table 6.1: Auto-immune hemolytic anemias

Warm antibodies	Cold antibodies
Primary	
Idiopathic AIHA	Chronic cold
AIHA + thrombocytopenia	hemagglutinin
(Evan's Syndrome)	disease
Secondary	
SLE	*Mycoplasma pneumoniae*
Lymphoma	*Infectious mononucleosis*
Chronic active hepatitis	Lymphoma
Ulcerative colitis	
Drugs	
Ovarian tumors	

Immunology. Most cold auto-antibodies are of the IgM class and of low avidity. They will cause the patient's red cells, once removed from the body, to agglutinate spontaneously when the temperature falls to room temperature or below. These antibodies are sometimes called cold agglutinins. Warm auto-antibodies can be screened for using the direct globulin test (direct Coombs test – Section 4.5.3). The direct Coombs test can, however, produce both false positive results (e.g. if infection or drugs have damaged the red cells leading to non-specific binding of protein) and false negative results (e.g. because it is unable to detect complement on the red cells). Further information can be gained by testing the patient's serum both undiluted and with complement added against untreated and enzyme-treated panels of red cells of different blood groups. Warm auto-antibodies are usually of the IgG class and directed against the Rhesus antigen complex.

Immunopathology. The site of destruction of the red cells in AIHA depends on whether enough complement is fixed to cause lysis within the circulation. If IgG is bound to the red cell then the antibody coating will promote phagocytosis by macrophages, mainly within the spleen. Continuous exposure of the spleen to abnormal red cells leads to splenic enlargement.

Clinical features. The presenting features are those of anemia (fatigue, weakness, shortness of breath). Because of the increased red cell turnover the patient may become mildly jaundiced (bilirubin is a breakdown product of heme). The spleen may be slightly enlarged. A careful search must be made for an underlying condition such as SLE, chronic lymphocytic leukemia or viral infections.

Treatment. The initial choice is high dose prednisolone. If this fails then splenectomy may be considered followed by immunosuppression. The condition usually resolves spontaneously eventually.

6.2.3 Idiopathic thrombocytopenic purpura (ITP)

The first step in the coagulation (clotting) pathway is the adhesion of platelets (thrombocytes) to the damaged part of the blood vessel. These platelets become 'sticky' and aggregate helping to breach small defects. They also release arachidonic acid and various other substances which promote the functioning of the clotting cascade. Any defect in platelet quality or quantity will lead to easy bruising or spontaneous bleeding. Purpura is the name given to the small bruises (each about the size of a match-head) which appear under the surface of the skin in platelet deficiency states.

Epidemiology. Thrombocytopenic purpura may occur alone (ITP) or as part of another disease (usually SLE). It may also occur as a complication of drug therapy. Most patients with ITP are young and female. In children ITP usually follows an acute viral infection.

Immunology. Ninety per cent of patients with ITP have IgG platelet auto-antibodies and 50% have IgM auto-antibodies. Auto-antibodies coat the platelets and lead to their premature destruction by macrophages predominantly in the spleen.

Clinical features. The onset is usually sudden. The patient develops widespread purpura. There may also be bleeding from other sites, for example, the nose, the gut or the uterus. Occasionally brain hemorrhage leads to death. The infants of affected women frequently have ITP at birth which resolves after a few weeks.

Associated diseases. The co-existence of ITP and AIHA is called Evan's Syndrome.

Treatment. The disease often remits spontaneously. Patients with severe bleeding or a very low platelet count are treated with steroids. If steroids fail to control the situation a splenectomy is performed. Intravenous gamma-globulin is an effective treatment but the benefit is often transient. It may thus be useful pre-operatively or to cover delivery.

6.3 Endocrine system: thyroid disease

Under normal circumstances the thyroid gland produces two iodine-containing hormones, thyroxine (T4) and tri-iodothyronine (T3), which play a major role in controlling the body's metabolic rate. T4 and T3 are stored within the thyroid as thyroglobulin (TG) and are released in response to another hormone, thyroid-stimulating hormone (TSH) produced by the anterior pituitary gland. The rate of TSH release is controlled by thyrotrophin-releasing hormone (TRH) which is secreted by the hypothalamus. Both TRH and TSH secretion are under negative feedback control (see *Figure 6.2*).

Auto-antibodies have been described directed against TG, the TSH receptor on the thyrocyte and intracytoplasmic antigens (thyroid peroxidase antibodies) (see Section 3.1.3). Autoimmune thyroid disease is a family of common disorders of thyroid function.

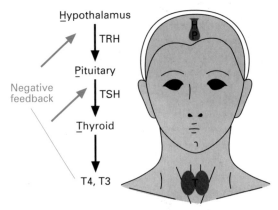

Figure 6.2: *Control of thyroid hormones.*

6.3.1 Grave's Disease (thyrotoxicosis)

Grave's Disease is the most common cause of hyperthyroidism. Robert Grave was a Dublin physician (1786–1853).

Immunology. Grave's Disease results from thyroid stimulation by TSH receptor antibodies. The TSH receptor comprises two sub-units linked by a disulfide bond. Most TSH receptor antibodies bind to the same part of the receptor molecule as TSH itself. However, antibodies vary in their affinity for the site. TSH receptor antibodies demonstrate light-chain restriction in the majority of patients with Grave's Disease.

When these antibodies bind to the TSH receptor they initiate the secretion of T3 and T4 in the same way that TSH itself would do.

Immunopathology. The thyroid gland becomes diffusely enlarged. The gland is very vascular and infiltrated with lymphocytes and plasma cells. The follicles of the gland also enlarge and are filled with colloid. The thyroid cells show a high frequency of MHC class II expression. Thyrocyte class II expression can be induced by TSH, TSH receptor antibodies and by cytokines.

Clinical features. There are four cardinal groups of features in Grave's Disease: goiter, hyperthyroidism, eye signs and indurated skin changes (*Figure 6.3*).

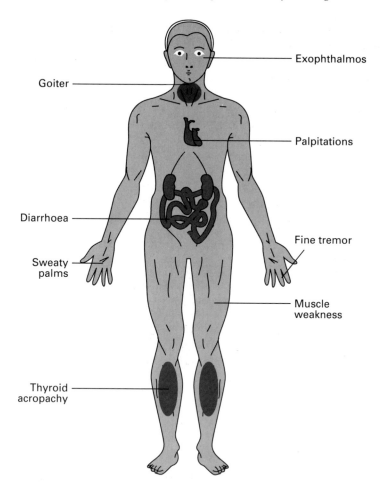

Figure 6.3: *Clinical features of Grave's Disease.*

The thyroid is situated anteriorly in the neck. As it enlarges the swelling may first become palpable and then clearly visible (a goiter). Large goiters may cause symptoms as a result of pressure of the enlarged gland on the trachea. Because of its increased vascularity, blood flow (a bruit) through the gland can often be heard through a stethoscope applied over the gland.

Excess production of T4 and T3 has an effect on almost all organs in the body. The commonest symptoms of hyperthyroidism are weight loss (usually with a good appetite), nervousness, increased sweating, intolerance of the heat, palpitations and a rapid pulse, and diarrhea. The principal signs of hyperthyroidism include a rapid pulse which may be irregular. The rapid heart rate and high cardiac output may lead to cardiac failure. The skin feels hot and moist and there is commonly a fine tremor of the outstretched hands. The patient is often restless and unable to settle to anything. Despite an apparent abundance of energy the patient may tire very easily. Muscle weakness is common, particularly of the proximal muscles (the limb muscles nearest the trunk). The patient is unable to stand from a crouched position unaided.

Retraction of the upper eyelid, so that a rim of white sclera can be seen above the colored iris, is common in all forms of hyperthyroidism. Similarly a phenomenon called 'lid lag' occurs in which movement of the upper eyelid lags behind that of the eyeball when the patient is asked to look downwards. In addition to these eye signs some patients with Grave's Disease develop an infiltrative ophthalmopathy. This condition is unique to Grave's Disease. There is an increase in the volume of connective tissue behind the eyes and in the size of the external muscles which move the eye. This leads to protrusion of the eyeballs (exophthalmos) and weakness or paralysis of the eye muscles (ophthalmoplegia). If the exophthalmos is marked patients may be unable to close their eyes even when sleeping and so abrasions may occur. Asymmetrical exophthalmos may be associated with double vision. Involvement of the optic nerve may cause blindness. The mechanism underlying the infiltrative ophthalmopathy of Grave's disease is poorly understood. One suggestion is that TG travels in the lymphatics from the thyroid to the eye muscles and then evokes an immune response.

Some patients with Grave's Disease plus ophthalmopathy also develop indurative skin lesions. These are due to deposition of mucopolysaccharide in the skin of the lower leg leading to 'pretibial myxedema'. Rarely these skin lesions also occur elsewhere on the body.

Associated diseases. Many patients with Grave's Disease also have other ADs. For example, 1% develop myasthenia gravis and 3% develop PA.

Prognosis. The course of untreated Grave's Disease is variable. In many patients the severity of hyperthyroidism is cyclic, sometimes going into prolonged or temporary remission. Ultimately a large proportion of patients develop hypothyroidism.

Treatment. There are three approaches to the treatment of Grave's Disease: medical, surgical and with radioactive iodine. Medical treatment consists of administering drugs which inhibit the synthesis of T4 and T3. A course of treatment usually lasts 12–18 months. However, over 50% of patients relapse and the drugs are occasionally associated with serious side effects such as bone marrow suppression. Surgical removal of the majority of the thyroid gland is the treatment of choice in patients with more than one relapse after medical treatment, or in those with a large goiter. Radioactive iodine is used in those considered unfit for surgery or in those over child-bearing age. There is a high frequency of hypothyroidism after all these forms of treatment and so patients should have their thyroid function checked every 1–2 years or if symptoms develop.

The eye disease of Grave's Disease does not always respond to treatment of the underlying thyroid disease. It may be necessary to give large doses of steroids (Section 7.5.1) if discomfort is marked or vision threatened. Alternatively, the orbit can be decompressed surgically.

Genetics. Grave's Disease is weakly associated with DR3. Associations have also been demonstrated between T cell receptor (TCR) genes and Grave's Disease. Increased frequencies of particular polymorphisms of TCR C_β and TCR $V\alpha$ have been reported.

6.3.2 Hashimoto's thyroiditis

Hashimoto's thyroiditis is often regarded as the prototype of organ-specific AD. It is the most common cause of hypothyroidism. Other causes include congenital enzyme deficiency, pituitary failure and neck surgery.

Immunology. Hashimoto's thyroiditis is associated with auto-antibodies to TG and thyroid peroxidase antibodies (previously called thyroid microsomal antibodies). TG is a glycoprotein dimer that is secreted by the thyrocyte into the colloid and then into the circulation (Section 3.1.3). Up to 15% of the normal population has TG auto-antibodies. They may belong to the IgG1, IgG2 or IgG4 sub-class and bind to a variety of epitopes. IgG1 TG antibodies may be able to fix complement and attract killer cells to the thyroid target cell.

Thyroid peroxidase (TPO) is required for the coupling reaction that yields T4 and T3 (Section 3.1.3). TPO auto-antibodies are found in low titers in 20% of the normal population and in high titers in most patients with Hashimoto's thyroiditis. It is unlikely that either TG or TPO auto-antibodies are directly involved in the etiology of autoimmune thyroiditis as they are usually polyclonal and directed at more than one epitope. Nevertheless, like TG auto-antibodies, IgG1 sub-class TPO antibodies can fix complement and lyse thyroid cells.

Immunopathology. The thyroid gland is usually enlarged. There is diffuse lymphocytic infiltration with obliteration of thyroid follicles and fibrosis. The infiltrate is mainly of T cells. In general CD4 cells predominate in areas of dense lymphoid aggregates, whereas CD8 cells predominate elsewhere.

Clinical features. Hashimoto's thyroiditis may present as a goiter, as hypothyroidism, or both.

Hypothyroidism results in a slowing down of all the body's functions because of a deficiency of T4 and T3. It is often associated with a deposition of mucopolysaccharide below the skin (myxedema). The onset may be very insidious and so diagnosis can be difficult. The most common symptoms of hypothyroidism are weight gain, intolerance of the cold, muscle and joint pains, constipation and heavy menstrual periods (*Figure 6.4*). The skin becomes dry, cold and thickened. The hair is often coarse and brittle and there may be some balding. The facial features may alter and the voice become deeper. The pulse is slow and, particularly in the elderly, angina is a common consequence.

All mental processes are slowed. The patient may develop frank psychiatric features (myxedema madness) or lapse into unconsciousness (myxedema coma). Myxedema coma has a mortality rate, even when treated, of 50%.

Treatment. Hypothyroidism is treated by the oral administration of thyroxine. Treatment must be started with very low doses and built up slowly, especially in the elderly, because it is dangerous to speed up the body's metabolic rate suddenly.

6.3.3 Primary hypothyroidism

Primary hypothyroidism is the name given to spontaneous hypothyroidism in the absence of a goiter. It probably represents the end result of autoimmune thyroiditis.

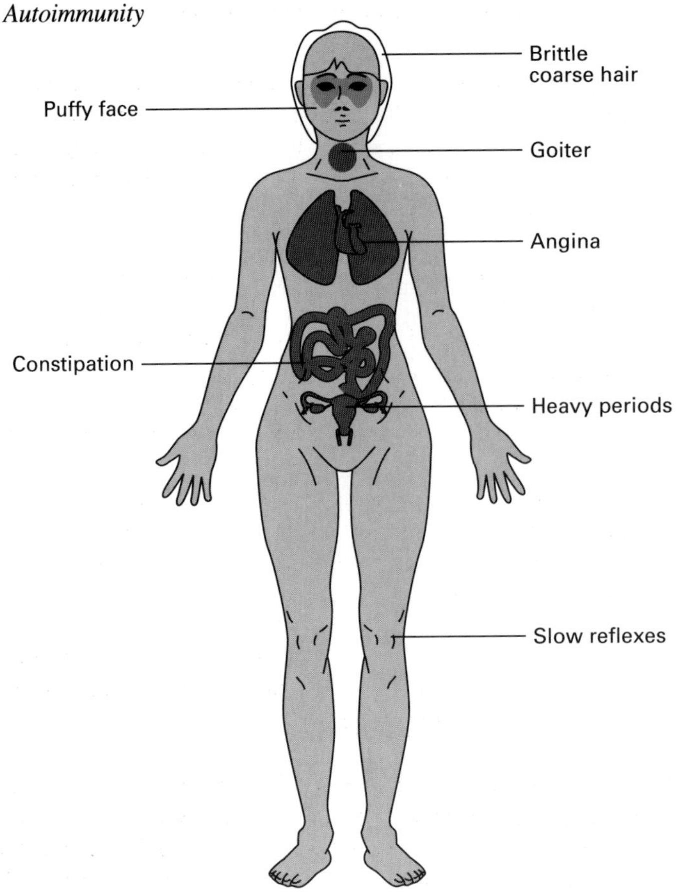

Figure 6.4: *Clinical features of hypothyroidism.*

Eighty per cent of patients have auto-antibodies to TG or TPO. The thyroid gland is small and fibrotic.

6.3.4 Type I-diabetes mellitus

Diabetes mellitus results from an inability to metabolize glucose adequately. There are two major types of diabetes. Type I (TI-DM) nearly always occurs before the age of 30 and is associated with an absolute dependence on exogenous insulin. Type II occurs in older people and is associated with obesity. It can usually be managed by dietary control and oral medication. TI-DM is an AD, Type II is not. There are peaks of onset of TI-DM in autumn and spring, suggesting a viral etiology.

Immunology. Over 90% of patients have circulating antibodies to the islet cells in the pancreas (which produce insulin) within the first month of diagnosis. The prevalence of these antibodies tends to decrease with time. A small group (about 10%) have persistent islet cell antibodies. They are likely to have other auto-antibodies and to develop other ADs. About 5% of patients also have insulin receptor antibodies.

Immunopathology. Early in the disease the pancreatic islet cells can be shown to express class II antigens and the islets have a heavy lymphocyte infiltrate. Late in the disease the islets shrivel and the inflammation disappears. The prolonged aberration in glucose metabolism produces a variety of secondary pathological changes which are beyond the scope of this book to describe.

Clinical features. A deficiency of insulin results in hyperglycemia. This in turn is associated with abnormalities of lipid metabolism and glycosylation of various tissues. These latter changes are responsible for many of the late complications of TI-DM. In the short term, a high blood sugar spills into the urine causing polyuria, thirst and dehydration. The patient may lapse into coma and die, either directly due to the hyperosmolar effect of the sugar or due to the ketoacidosis secondary to alternative routes of metabolism.

Long-term complications of DM include thickening of the vascular basement membrane producing retinal and renal changes; increased atheroma producing heart attacks and strokes; damage of nerves producing numbness of hands and feet; and sugar deposition in the lens producing cataracts.

Treatment. The aims of treatment are to mimic normal glucose metabolism by a combination of dietary manipulation and insulin administration. The means of achieving this aim are constantly improving.

Genetics. TI-DM is associated with a number of class I and II antigens. Family studies have conclusively demonstrated linkage between the HLA region and this disease. The majority of class I HLA antigens associated with TI-DM can be explained by their linkage disequilibrium with either DR3 or DR4. Over 95% of patients have either DR3 or DR4 or both. There is also a higher than expected frequency of DR3/DR4 heterozygotes in the patients suggesting that two different diabetogenic genes are involved. A negative association between DR2 and TI-DM has been found, indicating that this allele may be protective. (All negative associations have to be treated with caution as, when one or more allele are at raised frequency in a panel of patients, the remaining antigens in the allelic series have to be reduced in compensation. The overall gene frequency must always add up to 100%.)

The DR4 TI-DM patients are usually also DQw8-positive (DR4 can be associated with either DQw7 or DQw8) suggesting that this DQ allele may be a disease susceptibility gene. Another interpretation of DQ involvement in TI-DM has been put forward: resistance to TI-DM has been correlated with the presence of an aspartic acid residue at position 57 of the DQB chain. Consequently, susceptibility to the disease is associated with having any other amino acid at this position. This is consistent with the DQw8 association as this allele does not have an aspartic acid at codon 57 whereas DQw7 does.

The situation regarding the involvement of DQ in TI-DM susceptibility/resistance awaits confirmation and studies of TI-DM in Oriental populations have shown associations with DQ alleles having an aspartic acid at position 57 of DQB.

6.3.5 Autoimmune Addison's Disease

Autoimmune Addison's Disease is a condition leading to insufficiency of the adrenal glands. These glands, situated just above the kidneys, normally produce two main types of hormone – glucocorticoids, which play a role in sodium and glucose homeostasis, and mineralocorticoids, which are important in sodium homeostasis. The glucocorticoids play an essential role in the body's response to stress such as infection or surgery.

Immunology. Antibodies directed against the adrenal cortex are found in approximately 75% of women and 80% of men with autoimmune Addison's Disease. These auto-antibodies are directed against microsomes in the secretory cells of the three layers of the adrenal cortex. In addition, many patients also have auto-antibodies to gastric parietal cells, intrinsic factor and thyroid components. ANAs are, however, seldom found.

Clinical features. Patients with adrenal failure present with weight loss, postural hypotension (a fall in blood pressure on standing), weakness and excess pigmentation, especially in skin creases, scars and inside the mouth. The increased pigmentation occurs because the pituitary produces large amounts of ACTH (adrenocorticotrophic hormone) in an effort to stimulate the adrenal gland. ACTH and MSH (melanocyte stimulating hormone) have a common precursor molecule in the pituitary and have to be produced in equal quantities. It is the MSH which probably produces the pigmentation. If the patient encounters a stressful situation such as an intercurrent infection an Addisonian crisis may supervene. In this the patient collapses with a very low blood pressure and may die.

Genetics. Autoimmune Addison's Disease is associated with HLA-B8, DR3.

Treatment. Addison's Disease is treated with lifelong steroid replacement therapy.

6.3.6 Idiopathic hypoparathyroidism

The four parathyroid glands are situated in the neck; one at each pole of the thyroid gland. They secrete parathyroid hormone (PTH) which plays a major role in maintaining serum calcium levels. In hypoparathyroidism reduced secretion of PTH leads to hypocalcemia. The commonest cause of hypothyroidism is surgical removal of the glands, but rarely the disease occurs spontaneously. Idiopathic hypoparathyroidism is thought to be an autoimmune condition for two reasons: patients often (38%) have circulating auto-antibodies to parathyroid tissue, and the condition often occurs in association with other ADs, especially PA and Addison's Disease. The parathyroid glands in idiopathic hypoparathyroidism are atrophied and infiltrated with lymphocytes. The patient, who is usually young, presents with neuromuscular irritability manifested by muscle spasm, fits or abnormal heart rhythm. The condition is often associated with refractory infection of the skin with the yeast *Candida*. The low serum calcium is treated with vitamin D or its metabolites.

6.3.7 Infertility (some forms)

Primary ovarian failure. Primary ovarian failure may be associated with auto-antibodies directed against cells in the ovary. These auto-antibodies cross-react with cells in the adrenal cortex. Ovarian failure leads to absent menstruation and infertility.

Anti-sperm immunity. Some men develop antibodies against various sperm antigens resulting in reduced fertility. The reduced fertility is thought to be related to a reduction in sperm mobility due to coating with antibody.

Table 6.2: *Autoimmune polyglandular syndromes*

Type I	Type II
Hypoparathyroidism	Thyrotoxicosis
Addison's Disease	Hypothyroidism
Chronic active hepatitis	Type I-diabetes mellitus
Vitiligo	Addison's Disease
Pernicious anemia	Myasthenia gravis
Hypothyroidism	Celiac disease
	Pernicious anemia
	Vitiligo

6.3.8 Autoimmune polyendocrinopathies

A number of syndromes exists where the patient has AD of more than one endocrine gland. The two most common groups of associations are called type I and type II autoimmune polyglandular syndromes (*Table 6.2*). Type I (Blizzard's Syndrome) mainly affects children. The essential triad is idiopathic hypoparathyroidism, autoimmune Addison's Disease and chronic mucocutaneous candidiasis. Other associations are listed in *Table 6.2*. There are no known HLA associations with Type I. In contrast the more common type II (Schmidt–Carpenter Syndrome) is associated with the HLA-A1, B8, DR3 haplotype. It should be noted that there are other AD associated with this haplotype (e.g. SLE, SS) which are not part of the type II polyglandular syndrome.

Two other autoimmune associations are worthy of mention. The first is the association between insulin-resistant diabetes mellitus and the skin condition acanthosis nigricans. The insulin resistance is due to anti-insulin receptor antibodies. The second is the so-called POEMS syndrome (plasma cell dysplasia with polyneuropathy, organomegaly, endocrinopathy, M protein and skin changes). The endocrinopathy referred to is diabetes mellitus and failure of the gonads (70% of patients).

6.4 Skin

6.4.1 Pemphigus vulgaris

Pemphigus vulgaris is a blistering condition affecting both the mucous membranes and the skin. The blisters are within the epidermis. Some cases of pemphigus are drug-induced (e.g. penicillamine, captopril).

Immunology. Ninety per cent of patients have circulating IgG antibodies to squamous epithelial cell surface. The titer of antibody fluctuates with disease severity. These antibodies produce pemphigus-like lesions if injected into monkey skin.

Immunopathology. The earliest pathological lesion seems to be dissolution of intercellular bridges in the epidermis. Direct immunofluorescence of perilesional skin shows IgG antibodies, C1q, C3, C4, properdin and factor B in the intercellular space.

Clinical features. The condition begins with oral ulceration. Then the patient develops widespread flaccid, weepy large blisters (bullae). The blisters are superficial and quickly burst. The skin at the edge of the lesions can easily be dislodged by sliding pressure (Nikolsky sign). Remission of the disease is rare and it is rapidly fatal unless large doses of corticosteroids are administered. Immunosuppressants are usually required in addition. If the patient survives, treatment can be withdrawn after 2–3 years.

Genetics. There is a very strong association between DR4 and pemphigus vulgaris in the Ashkenaze Jewish population. These DR4 patients have the Dw10 DR4 subtype and no other DR4 Dw variant is found. Other studies have implicated DR6 with the disease. DNA sequence homology between these alleles is found within the third hypervariable region of $DR\beta_1$, suggesting that a shared DR epitope may confer susceptibility to this disease.

6.4.2 Bullous pemphigoid

This disease is about twice as common as pemphigus. The blisters are below the epidermis and so less likely to burst.

Immunology. Seventy-five per cent of patients have circulating antibodies to basement membrane zone antigens. The antibodies will not produce lesions in monkey skin. Their titer does not vary with disease activity.

Immunopathology. Direct immunofluorescence of perilesional skin shows deposition of IgG and C3 as a continuous band along the basement membrane layer.

Clinical features. The blisters often begin around an old scar. They tend to be dense and dome shaped, and often contain blood. Mucous membrane ulcers are rare. The lesions can be controlled by moderate doses of corticosteroids and the disease usually goes into remission after about a year.

6.4.3 Dermatitis herpetiformis

Dermatitis herpetiformis is an autoimmune condition associated with small vesicles on the skin.

Immunology. Twenty-five per cent of patients have circulating antibodies to reticulin.

Immunopathology. Direct immunofluorescence of uninvolved skin shows deposition of IgA. In 85% of patients the IgA is deposited in a granular fashion at the tips of the dermal papillae. In the remainder the deposits are linear along the entire basement membrane. Most patients have bowel pathology indistinguishable from celiac disease (Section 6.1.3) which is usually symptomless.

Clinical features. These small blisters, which are extremely itchy, occur in crops predominantly on the elbows, knees, buttocks, neck and shoulder. The severity waxes and wanes but the condition seldom goes into prolonged remission. A gluten-free diet leads to improvement but may take up to 2 years to work. As in celiac disease there is an increased risk of intestinal lymphoma.

Genetics. The same genetic associations exist as for celiac disease (Section 6.1.3)

6.4.4 Vitiligo

Vitiligo is a common autoimmune condition. The pigment containing cells of the skin (melanocytes) are completely destroyed, often in a patchy distribution. The resulting patchy depigmentation is more noticeable in dark skinned patients. It usually begins over the knuckles. The face and neck are frequently affected and the depigmentation is asymmetrical. In about one-third of patients spontaneous recovery occurs. In itself the condition is of no significance but it is associated with other autoimmune disorders; most commonly TI-DM, PA, Addison's Disease or autoimmune thyroid disease.

6.5 Neuromuscular system

6.5.1 Multiple sclerosis

Multiple sclerosis (MS) is a common disease of the central nervous system. It is caused by plaques of demyelination which spare the neurones and their axonal sheaths. These plaques are disseminated not only in place but also in time.

Epidemiology. The most intriguing feature about the epidemiology of MS is that its prevalence varies with latitude. With the exception of Japan (where the prevalence is low), prevalence is positively correlated with distance from the equator in both hemispheres. The highest prevalence is recorded in Orkney and the Shetland Isles. Studies of migrants shed further light on this observation. Immigrants to the U.K. from the Indian subcontinent, the West Indies and Africa have a low risk of MS, but their children, born in the U.K., have the same risk as other U.K. residents. These, and other observations, provide evidence that MS is due to an exogenous agent present in cooler climates which is acquired in childhood. Many viruses, including measles and retroviruses, have been implicated as this exogenous agent but the evidence is inconclusive. Onset of the disease before the age of 15 and after the age 55 is rare.

Genetics. A genetic influence in MS has been suspected for many years. First degree relatives have a 10–15 times increased risk of developing MS. The HLA association is with HLA-DR2 and with the haplotype A3, B7, CW7, DW2.

Immunology. There are no circulating auto-antibodies associated with MS and so some have questioned whether it can truly be regarded as an AD. However, the condition is confined to the central nervous system and the cerebrospinal fluid in MS has increased levels of IgG with oligoclonal bands. A small portion of the oligoclonal immunoglobulin reacts with myelin basic protein. Thus there may be local production of auto-antibody within the brain. Patients with MS have abnormal T suppressor cell function.

Immunopathology. In early lesions there are inflammatory changes with mononuclear infiltration. Older lesions have plasma cells and lymphocytes within them. In later stages there is glial scarring (i.e. sclerosis).

Clinical features. The plaques of MS may occur anywhere in the central nervous system but are predominantly in the white matter of the brain. They have a predilection for the optic nerves, the areas around the ventricles of the brain, the brain stem and the upper spinal cord. The clinical features of an individual patient will depend on the positioning of the plaques. Generally the disease begins with a single symptom. The most common presenting features are blurred vision, double vision, numbness or tingling, or muscle weakness. The patient often makes a complete recovery from the initial attack. Subsequent attacks occur unpredictably and usually leave some residual disability. Thus the patient may become progressively more disabled as the disease continues. Common features of established MS are unsteady gait, loss of bladder control, an altered mental state (e.g. euphoria), paralysis and altered sensation.

The course of the disease is very variable. The average life expectancy from onset is 20–30 years. Patients likely to do badly include those with an onset after the age of 40, those with a progressive course from the start, those who relapse early, those with a family history of MS and those of lower social class.

Many different treatments have been tried in MS including dietary manipulation, the use of hyperbaric oxygen and immunosuppression. In such an unpredictable disease with natural remissions, it is hard to evaluate therapy. To date there is no treatment which has been shown conclusively to alter the course of MS, although steroids may shorten the duration of relapses.

6.5.2 Myasthenia gravis

Myasthenia gravis (MG) is an AD of the neuromuscular junction which is characterized by abnormal muscle fatigability. Each muscle fiber in skeletal muscle is supplied by a single nerve fiber. The area where the message is transmitted from nerve to muscle is the motor end plate, and the gap between the nerve and the muscle is called a synapse. The electrical impulse which arises at the nerve ending results in the release of a chemical messenger, acetylcholine. This chemical diffuses across the synapse and attaches to specific acetylcholine receptors (AChR) on the muscle fiber. This in turn opens up ionic channels in the muscle leading to depolarization. In MG auto-antibodies to the AChR block the action of the chemical transmitter.

Epidemiology. MG occurs in all races and all age groups. The most common onset is in early adult life. Clustering within families is rare but within the individual patient it is often associated with Graves's Disease and less commonly with RA, SLE or

TI-DM. MG may also be precipitated by treatment with certain drugs. The most common of these is penicillamine. Fifteen per cent of patients with MG have an associated tumor in the thymus (a thymoma).

Genetics. MG is associated with the haplotype A1, B8, CW7, C4AQO, C4B1, Bfs, DR3.

Immunology. Ninety per cent of patients with MG have circulating antibodies to the AChR (Section 3.1.3). The antibody binds to the AChR which is then endocytosed. Thus the neuromuscular junction becomes depleted of receptors. However, the titer of AChR antibody does not correlate with the severity of the disease. This can be explained by the fact that the AChR is heterogeneous and that auto-antibodies may have varying affinity for it. Patients with MG also frequently have ANAs, anti-thyroid antibodies and antibodies to striated muscle.

Immunopathology. The main pathological abnormalities in MG are found, not in muscle, but in the thymus. Eighty per cent of patients have either thymic hyperplasia with germinal center formation (65%) or true thymomas (15%). The latter are more common in young women.

Clinical features. The earliest feature is of muscle weakness after repetitive use. The muscles first affected are usually the muscles which move the eye and so the patient complains of double vision or drooping eyelids. Later the proximal muscles may become involved leading to difficulty in rising from a chair, problems in climbing stairs or combing hair. Later still there may be difficulty in holding up the head or swallowing. Before the advent of modern treatment the mortality of the disease was 25%. About the same proportion go into spontaneous remission.

The drug treatment for MG consists of giving anticholinesterases. These drugs increase the availability of acetylcholine. The majority of patients benefit from surgical removal of the thymus. In patients who fail to respond to either of these maneuvers immunosuppression is often effective.

Approximately one in seven babies born to women with MG will have neonatal myasthenia due to transfer of maternal antibodies. This condition lasts for about 3 months and then resolves completely.

6.6 Conclusion

Autoimmune disease may occur in almost every major organ system. In many of these diseases cellular autoimmunity predominates: the organ is infiltrated with lymphocytes and rendered permanently non-functional. The autoimmune process then 'burns out' as there is no tissue remaining for attack. In other diseases antibody-mediated autoimmunity is the major abnormality. The activity is these diseases may wax and wane and, occasionally, disappear altogether.

Further reading

Eisenbarth, G. S. (1986) Type I diabetes mellitus. *New Engl. J. Med.,* **314**, 1360

O'Connor, G. and Davies, T F. (1990) Human autoimmune thyroid disease. A mechanistic update. *Trends Endocrinol.,* **1**. 266

Rose, N. and Mackay, I (1985) *Autoimmune Diseases.* Academic Press, London.

Weatherall, D.J., Ledingham, J.G.G. and Warrell, D.A. (1987) *Oxford Textbook of Medicine.* Oxford University Press, Oxford.

7

LONG TERM PROGNOSIS AND TREATMENT OF AUTOIMMUNE DISEASES

Prognosis

7.1 Prognosis of autoimmune diseases

The prognosis of ADs is very variable. Some, like pemphigus are life-threatening and have a very high mortality if not treated. Others, like vitiligo are of nuisance value only. Some, like AIHA are self-limiting. Others such as RA and Sjögren's Syndrome last for the rest of the patient's life. The autoimmune component of many of the organ-specific ADs appears to be self-limiting. For example, islet antibodies are only seen at the onset of T1-DM. However, it may be that once the target organ (e.g. the thyroid, the pancreatic islet) has been destroyed that auto-antigen is no longer expressed and so the stimulus for the autoimmune process is removed. The patients, however, have to contend with a non-functioning organ for the rest of their lives.

Most of the chronic ADs follow a relapsing and remitting course. This is particularly true for RA, SLE, myasthenia gravis and multiple sclerosis. Relapses may appear to occur spontaneously or may be triggered by intercurrent viral infections or by stress. There is considerable interest as to whether dietary manipulation may help to prolong remission in these diseases. Pregnancy may also have a profound effect on the activity of these diseases. Most patients with RA go into remission during pregnancy although there is often a marked flare post-partum. In contrast patients with SLE may have more active disease during pregnancy. Flares in SLE may also be precipitated by high-estrogen oral contraceptive pills and by exposure to ultraviolet radiation.

All chronic ADs are associated with a reduced life expectancy. In PBC and CAH most premature deaths are due to liver failure. In RA deaths from most causes occur earlier than expected, although deaths from infection are especially common. Increased deaths from infection are also seen in SLE. Renal involvement is the commonest cause of death which can be directly attributed to the disease process in SLE. On the whole the loss of life expectancy in both SLE and RA is related to the cumulative disease activity. Patients with mild disease not requiring hospital referral have a normal life span. RA is estimated to shorten life expectancy by between 3 and 18 years depending on disease severity.

7.2 Malignant transformation in autoimmune disease

The ultimate consequence of chronic stimulation and activation of the immune system may be malignant transformation. All ADs are associated with immune hyperactivity and there is evidence of an increased incidence of tumors of the immune system (also called lympho-proliferative malignancies) in many ADs (*Table 7.1*).

Table 7.1: *The association between AD and malignancy*

Autoimmune disease	Type of tumor	Site of presentation	Relative risk
Sjögren's Syndrome	NHL	Parotid Lymph nodes	44
Hashimoto's thyroiditis	NHL	Thyroid gland Lymph nodes	67
RA	NHL	Lymph nodes	10
Celiac disease	NHL Carcinoma	Small intestine Esophagus	
Scleroderma	Broncho-alveolar carcinoma	Lung	4
Pernicious anemia	Carcinoma	Stomach	4

NHL = non-Hodgkin's lymphoma.

The highest risk of malignant transformation is seen in patients with SS (Section 5.11). Patients with SS develop non-Hodgkin's lymphoma up to 44 times more commonly than the general population. The latent period between the onset of SS and the development of the malignancy may be up to 20 years. The tumors are usually monoclonal B-cell malignancies and they usually develop either in the salivary glands or in the lymph nodes.

Hashimoto's thyroiditis (Section 6.3.2) is sometimes complicated by the development of a malignant lymphoma in the thyroid gland. These patients may also develop lymphomas outside the thyroid gland, mainly in lymph nodes. Similar tumors also occur with increased frequency in RA and in diabetes. A number of explanations have been put forward for this association between AD and malignancy. They are:

(a) That both conditions are due to the same forbidden clone of lymphocytes. This theory suggests that AD is a secondary phenomenon – the rapid turnover of tumor cells allows mutation to form cell lines which can react immunologically against normal cells.

(b) That the patient has an innate or acquired susceptibility to both AD and immune malignancy. This susceptibility might have a genetic basis or be due to a common causative agent such as the Epstein–Barr virus (Section 3.2.3).

(c) That chronic activation of the immune system leads in some cases to malignant transformation.

(d) That treatment of the AD produces the malignancy.

(e) That the association is due to chance.

In the current light of knowledge explanation (c) fits best with the observed facts.

Association with other malignancies is also seen in AD (see *Table 7.1*). In addition malignancy may be associated with development of autoimmune phenomena. For example, patients with chronic lymphocytic leukemia often develop auto-antibodies or even overt AD.

Treatment

Treatment of the ADs may be divided into four broad categories: specific replacement therapy; disease modifying therapy; non-specific immunosuppressive therapy; and experimental immunomodulation.

7.3 Specific therapy

Many organ-specific ADs are associated with organ destruction and malfunction. Fortunately in many instances it is possible to replace the missing products of the defective organ, for instance by giving thyroxine in Hashimoto's thyroiditis, insulin in TI-DM, by artificial tears and saliva in Sjögren's Syndrome, vitamin B12 in PA and so on.

7.4 Disease modifying therapies

In multi-system AD and in organ-specific AD where inflammation plays a prominent role, often the only avenue of treatment is to try and dampen down the inappropriate immune response. Two groups of drugs have been identified which have some effect on the immune response. The first group are the so-called disease modifying drugs used predominantly in the rheumatic diseases, and the second group are the immunosuppressive drugs which are discussed in the next section. The disease modifying drugs are listed in *Table 7.2*. These drugs appear to have some action on the underlying disease process rather than being simply symptomatic therapy. Their exact mode of action is unknown; indeed they probably each have a different mode of action. They were discovered by serendipity. Gold injections were used in the 1920s to treat tuberculosis. They were introduced in the treatment of RA in 1934 because RA was thought to resemble a chronic mycobacteria infection. The infective theory for RA has now largely been discounted – but gold still works! Similarly sulfasalazine was manufactured in 1942 as a combination of two drugs, 5-aminosalicylic acid (an anti-inflammatory agent) and sulfapyridine (an antibiotic), because RA was thought to be an inflammatory arthritis due to a bacterial agent. Again, the infective theory is no longer held and it has been shown that 5-aminosalicylic acid is not absorbed from the gut – but sulfasalazine works! Disease modifying drugs share the following properties: they take several weeks to work, they have a high side-effect profile and they only work in a proportion of cases. Extensive immunological work has been done to try and establish how they work.

Gold compounds have been shown to have several properties which may explain their efficacy. *In vitro* gold compounds have been shown to interfere with the ability of macrophages to present antigen. This action leads to a diminished *in vitro* lymphocyte response to mitogens and antigens. Gold also has an effect on the complement pathway. It has been shown to block C1 activity and to prevent the formation of C3 convertase.

Table 7.2: *Disease-modifying drugs used in autoimmune diseases*

Disease	Drug
Rheumatoid arthritis	Intramuscular gold
	Oral gold
	D-Penicillamine
	Sulfasalazine
	Chloroquine
	Hydroxychloroquine
Systemic lupus erythematosus	Chloroquine
(skin and joint disease)	Hydroxychloroquine
Dermatitis herpetiformis	Dapsone

D-penicillamine inhibits the *in vitro* sulfhydryl-dependent heat denaturation of IgG. This suggests that it may prevent the formation of auto-antigenic IgG aggregation *in vitro*. It is also a potent inhibitor of myeloperoxidase activity and so may be able to protect tissues from damage by reactive oxygen species. D-penicillamine has an inhibitor effect on T helper function.

The anti-malarial drugs, chloroquine and hydroxychloroquine, appear to inhibit IL-1 production. They also have lysosomotropic properties. Chloroquine reduces prolactin levels and lymphocytes are known to have prolactin receptors.

The study of sulfasalazine is hampered by the fact that it has many metabolites, any one of which might be the active moiety of the drug. The parent compound and several metabolites have been shown to suppress lymphocyte response to various mitogens.

Successful treatment of patients with active RA with any of these compounds will be associated with a normalization of levels of circulating activated lymphocytes, and of abnormal lymphocyte function tests. Levels of rheumatoid factor and immunoglobulins often fall. These observations do not shed any light on the actual mode of action of the drugs, for a change in these tests towards normal may be an effect rather than a cause of the improved disease activity.

7.5 Immunosuppression

Some drugs are known to have a direct action on the immune system. Unfortunately in doing this it is impossible to avoid suppressing the patient's normal immune response at the same time. Thus immunosuppressive therapy is always associated with an increased risk of infection and sometimes with an increased cancer risk.

7.5.1 Corticosteroids

Cortisone was first used in the treatment of RA in 1949. The effects on the disease were dramatic but the initial enthusiastic use of steroids was replaced by disillusion in the late 1950s as the first reports of long-term side effects were published (high infection rate, obesity, thinning of the skin and bones, high blood pressure and steroid-induced diabetes). Thus steroids are now reserved for severe RA and for other ADs with severe complications (e.g. SLE, chronic active hepatitis, pemphigus). Synthetic analogs of cortisone have now been made which are more potent but have fewer side effects.

In low doses (less than 10 mg prednisolone per day) steroids have predominantly an anti-inflammatory effect. High doses of steroids (e.g. 1 g methylprednisolone) may have profound effects on the immune system. A single dose of a corticosteroid given orally or intravenously results in a reduction in the number of circulating lymphocytes, particularly T cells, at 4–6 hours. This is due to a redistribution of lymphocytes to peripheral lymph nodes and to bone marrow. The effect is seen to some extent with prednisolone doses as low as 5 mg but is profound after a pulse of methylprednisolone. The counts return to normal within 48 hours. During the period of lymphopenia those lymphocytes which remain in the circulation show a profoundly impaired response to mitogens. *In vivo* this effect may inhibit the movement of T lymphocytes to sites of antigen deposition.

High doses of steroids reduce circulating immunoglobulin levels even in normal individuals. They also affect monocyte distribution and function. Monocyte bactericidal activity is diminished. Steroids also prevent the release of IL-1 which, in turn influences the production of IL-2.

Steroids modulate a variety of cell functions by binding to cytoplasmic steroid receptors. The steroid–receptor complex then migrates into the cell nucleus and interacts with the non-histone nuclear protein of DNA. This results in the synthesis of RNA and new protein molecules. One such protein is lipocortin. Among other actions lipocortin inhibits phospholipase A activity. This in turn prevents the synthesis of prostaglandins, leukotrienes and platelet activating factor – all mediators of inflammation.

7.5.2 Cytotoxic drugs

The immunosuppressive/cytotoxic drugs fall into three main groups: alkylating agents, purine analogs and folic acid antagonists. Alkylating agents contain an alkyl radical substituted with one or more reactive end-groups, usually chlorine atoms. The principal drugs in this group are cyclophosphamide and chlorambucil. Both these drugs are activated in the liver to a compound which binds avidly to guanine bases in DNA. This leads to mismatching of base pairs during DNA synthesis and covalent cross-linking between the DNA strands of the double helix. This, in turn, prevents separation of the strands and so cell replication cannot occur and the cells die. B cells are more sensitive to cyclophosphamide than mature T cells, but less sensitive than precursors of suppressor T cells and amplifiers of suppressor cells.

The purine analogs are incorporated into DNA and RNA and interfere with nucleic acid synthesis. The chief purine analog used is azathioprine. It is rapidly converted in the intestinal wall to 6-mercaptopurine. Its effect on lymphocytes is dose dependent and related to concomitant steroid administration. Azathioprine has little effect on antibody production but does suppress T cell responses.

Folic acid antagonists bind to dihydrofolate reductase and prevent conversion of dihydrofolic acid to tetrafolic acid, a necessary step in DNA synthesis. Methotrexate is the representative drug. The *in-vitro* binding of methotrexate to dihydrofolate reductase is only slowly reversible and so the drug need only be administered once a week. It is widely used in the treatment of polymyositis and RA.

7.5.3 Cyclosporin A

Cyclosporin A, discovered in 1972, is a lipid-soluble polypeptide of 11 amino acids produced by two strains of fungi. It has marked immunosuppressive properties but, unlike the cytotoxic drugs, does not cause bone marrow depression. Instead, it acts predominantly on T helper cells. It passively crosses the cell surface membrane and binds to a cytoplasmic protein called cyclophilin. This protein is found in many cells including T cells. It then seems to work at the level of nuclear transcription. Lymphokine production, for example of IL-2, is inhibited and so cytotoxic T cells cannot be generated and T helper-cell-dependent responses are inhibited. Cyclosporin A is very effective in the prevention of transplantation rejection and, if given early, may delay the onset of insulin dependence in TI-DM. It has been used with moderate success in ITP, SLE, polymyositis, RA, myasthenia gravis and primary biliary cirrhosis. Cyclosporin A has a number of important side effects: it causes a reversible renal toxicity, hirsutism, gum hypertrophy, depression, anorexia, nausea and muscle tremors. Lymphoproliferative lesions which are polyclonal and related to EBV infection are also described.

7.6 Physical immunomodulation

Since the lymphocyte seems to be at the center of the autoimmune conundrum, one approach to therapy of these diseases, in severe cases, may be physically to deplete the patient of lymphocytes. This can be done by thoracic duct drainage, by lymphocytopheresis or by irradiation of lymphoid tissue. Alternatively the patient's plasma may be exchanged for fresh frozen plasma or plasma protein fraction, thus removing auto-antibodies. Plasma exchange is particularly beneficial in AIHA, myasthenia gravis and Goodpasture's Syndrome. Its role in SLE and RA is controversial. These treatments have all been shown to be effective but they are major undertakings and have considerable side effects.

7.7 Experimental immunotherapy

Unfortunately, immunosuppressive therapy is non-specific, leading to a reduction in all immune responses. Recent developments have opened the possibility of more specific therapy directed at the processes of immune recognition and regulatory responses. All these treatments are still in the experimental phase.

The immune response, whether autoreactive or not, is characterized by an antigen presenting cell (APC) offering a peptide (either foreign or of self origin) through its class II MHC molecules to the T cell receptor. If the T cell receptor has specificity for both self MHC and peptide antigen, and receives the necessary second signal, it will expand clonally and actively participate in the immune response. Theoretically, interference at any one of these three component levels (MHC, peptide or T cell recognition) should interrupt the immune response. This is summarized in *Figure 7.1*.

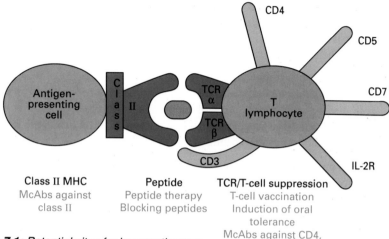

Class II MHC
McAbs against
class II

Peptide
Peptide therapy
Blocking peptides

TCR/T-cell suppression
T-cell vaccination
Induction of oral
tolerance
McAbs against CD4,
CD5, CD7, IL-2R, TCR

Figure 7.1: *Potential sites for immunotherapy.*

7.7.1 Antigen presentation and class II MHC

Removal or blocking of class II MHC on APCs should result in their inability to present peptide to the TCR. This can be achieved *in vitro* by using class II-specific monoclonal antibodies. If such antibodies were directed against class II framework epitopes (i.e. if they could recognize all class II molecules) they would block all antigen presentation and have an undesirable non-specific immunosuppressive effect. If a class II molecule is known to be associated with a particular disease, a more logical approach would be to use only highly-specific monoclonal antibodies to this antigen or epitope. As most individuals are heterozygous at each class II locus and as we all have multiple class II loci, the remaining class II molecules should be sufficient to present the multitude of foreign peptides which need to be recognized to maintain the integrity of the body.

Limited experimental work has been performed in animals, where class II monoclonal antibodies have been administered. The injection of antibodies to class II has a lethal effect on rhesus monkeys, although similar antibodies are tolerated by macaque monkeys. Any decision to use class II monoclonal antibodies, even in an engineered 'humanized' form, would be a courageous decision. Furthermore, any beneficial effect of such treatment would be dependent on continuous administration and it seems unlikely that such treatment offers a viable option.

7.7.2 Peptide therapy

A second possibility for therapeutic intervention is at the level of peptide binding to the class II molecule. Two approaches could be taken:

(a) If presentation of auto-antigen by a specific, associated HLA molecule is an important component of the disease process, the administration of an alternative peptide with high affinity for the class II antigen presenting groove, should displace and block the auto-antigen. There is considerable evidence that class II molecules can bind most peptides. However, some peptides have a high affinity for certain HLA specificities. If such a peptide could be found, which is also non-toxic, its use as a blocking agent could have great benefit. The peptide might, however, be immunogenic and circulating antibody could remove the blocking peptide before it bound to the class II molecule. The addition of sugars to peptides is one method being tried to reduce potential antigenicity.

(b) A second approach may come from the characterization of the immunological properties of the auto-antigen. There is some evidence that auto-antigens contain both disease-inducing and disease-suppressing epitopes. The latter may be responsible for inducing specific T cell suppression and if they can be identified and made synthetically, a therapeutic potential may exist.

Several problems apply to using peptide therapy. Some peptides have poor bioavailability, they often degrade easily and they are expensive. One possible alternative is to design non-peptide compound analogs which mimic the three-dimensional shape of blocking peptides.

Rational drug design. Rational drug design focuses on the creation of pharmaceutical compounds through detailed knowledge of their desired structure and their interaction with the biological target. This information can come from a variety of techniques such as X-ray crystallography, nuclear magnetic resonance, site-directed mutagenesis, epitope mapping and computer modeling of data obtained from antibody binding assays.

Antibody-directed drug design is based on the immune system's ability to recognize and produce antibodies to the three-dimensional structure of antigens, whether they are pharmacological receptors, enzymes or viruses. The antigen-combining sites of these antibodies are mirror images of the target's three-dimensional shape. By producing an anti-idiotype antibody, a positive image of the original target site can be made. Peptides can then be synthesized which are complementary to the anti-idiotype resulting in a receptor antagonist. The ultimate step is to construct a non-protein peptidomimetic compound which retains activity but can be administered orally. This can be achieved by the use of sophisticated computer-assisted drug design based on predictive three-dimensional spatial and charge characteristics, and also from crystallographic or nuclear magnetic resonance techniques.

Such work could be applied to the field of autoimmunity. If the epitopes which are critical within an HLA class II molecule or TCR associated with a particular AD can be deduced, it may be possible to design a compound which specifically interferes with this site and thus affect its ability to present or recognize a peptide implicated in the disease process.

7.7.3 Manipulation of T cell recognition and tolerance

Manipulation of T cell recognition and tolerance may be induced specifically through procedures such as T cell vaccination and induction of oral tolerance, or non-specifically by administration of monoclonal antibodies to T cell surface receptors.

T cell vaccination. T cell vaccination refers to the use of autoimmune T cells as vaccines to induce specific immunity to the T cells responsible for the disease. This area of research has largely been pioneered by Irun Cohen and his coworkers. More detailed explanations can be found elsewhere (Further reading, see Cohen (1980). Based on the observation that ADs are often slow to progress and may enter periods of complete or transient remission, they suggested that immune suppression, or the lack of it, may be an important aspect of control of AD. This was supported by observations from experimentally induced autoimmune conditions in animals where rapid progression may be followed by spontaneous remission.

Cohen's group isolated autoreactive T cell lines responding to myelin basic protein that could passively transfer experimental autoimmune encephalomyelitis (EAE) to naive animals. Animals surviving this procedure were subsequently resistant to further attempts at disease induction. Thus T cells could both transfer the condition and induce resistance. Whilst the disease can only be induced by viable, functionally active T cells, resistance can be induced by irradiated or attenuated T cells. The similarities of this phenomenon with that of vaccination against infectious disease has led to the term 'T cell vaccination'. The use of T cell vaccination to confer resistance has been demonstrated in a number of animal models of AD including adjuvant arthritis, experimental autoimmune thyroiditis, type II collagen arthritis and autoimmune neuritis. The protection mediated by T cell vaccination is specific and can only be induced by activated cells. Resting cells will neither passively transfer the disease nor confer resistance. This resistance is thought to be due to the generation of anti-idiotypic suppressor T cells.

Several clinical trials in humans are now under way. One such trial in RA uses T lymphocytes from synovial fluid exudates, expanded *in vitro* and then irradiated, to vaccinate patients. The outcome of these trials is awaited with interest.

Orally induced tolerance to auto-antigens. Orally induced tolerance to specific auto-antigens has been demonstrated in a number of animal models and has been shown significantly to modify AD. The main interface between the immune response and external antigens is at the level of mucosal surfaces. Of these the gut encounters the largest challenge with ingestion of food and bacterial antigens. However, these antigens rarely immunize and this pergastrically administered antigen usually induces a state of systemic hypoimmunoresponsiveness called oral tolerance. This observation provided the basis for experiments where auto-antigens were given orally and the effects on disease outcome were measured.

Feeding either rats or mice soluble type II collagen before giving the usual parenteral arthritogenic challenge of type II collagen has a significant effect. Fewer animals develop the arthritis and, in those who do, the onset is delayed. Similarly in a rat model for EAE, oral administration of myelin basic protein (MBP) before giving a standard MBP encephalitogenic challenge reduces both the incidence and severity of EAE. Oral administration of retinal S antigen can also prevent or diminish the severity of experimental autoimmune uveoretinitis in rats.

The induction of oral tolerance is dose dependent with larger doses giving increased levels of protection. This phenomenon is clearly specific, as feeding animals with an irrelevant antigen confers no protection in these animal models.

Oral administration of auto-antigen reduces the levels of both specific serum antibody and T cell responses, although neither is ever completely removed. In contrast, the levels of specific secretory IgA antibodies are usually increased. Experimental evidence indicates that oral tolerance occurs through regulatory T cell mechanisms. Passive transfer of oral tolerance can be achieved by injection of naive animals with CD8-positive splenic T cells taken from tolerant animals. Thus it is likely that these effects are induced by suppressor T cells.

A major difference between such animals and human AD is that the oral doses are given prior to disease onset whereas in the human situation the autoimmunity is already established. It is therefore possible that such treatment could exacerbate rather than improve the condition. A second consideration is that the patient may already be highly sensitized to the antigen being administered.

One strategy which has been suggested is that of using synthetic peptides or tolerogenic fragments of auto-antigens. This has an experimental basis as a non-encephalitogenic decapeptide of MBP can prevent EAE when given orally. An alternative approach may be to cross-link chemically or to modify the auto-antigen administered.

Evidence from an animal model of multiple sclerosis, chronic relapsing experimental allergic encephalomyelitis, has provided some encouragement for considering oral tolerance induction as a treatment in humans. Guinea pigs already suffering from this condition benefit considerably from MBP given orally, with the frequency and severity of subsequent relapses being diminished. This approach is now being evaluated in clinical trials. MBP is being administered orally to multiple sclerosis patients and type II collagen given in capsule form as a treatment for RA.

T cell monoclonal antibodies. Yet another approach may come from using monoclonal antibodies to T cell surface markers and receptors. Such antibodies are being used increasingly in bone marrow and renal transplantation patients and clinical trials of their efficacy in certain ADs are under way. Antibodies to a number of T cell surface components may have therapeutic potential. These include CD4, CD5, CD7, the receptor for IL-2, and the T cell receptor (either an α/β or γ/δ dimer).

The mode of action of these antibodies is not clear. Many fix complement and the reduction or removal of cells by cytotoxicity is likely. The down-regulation of T cell processes by these antibodies is also a possibility. Both mouse and rat monoclonal antibodies have been used in human clinical situations. However, these antibodies will need to be 'humanized' in order to avoid long-term sensitization of patients. Monoclonal antibodies to CD4 have been used to induce tolerance in bone marrow transplant patients. At least two centers are now testing anti-CD4 treatment in RA and prolonged remission in one patient has already been reported. Antibodies to CD7 have also been used in RA and, as CD5 antibodies are immunosuppressive *in vitro*, they may have potential clinically. Antibodies to the IL-2 receptor can inhibit immune responses and have been used in the treatment of bone marrow transplant patients. All of these antibody treatments induce non-specific immunosuppression. A potentially more specific approach would be to develop antibodies to T cell receptors. Every TCR represents a unique combination of TCR genes. If a particular TCR rearrangement is critical in recognizing a disease-specific auto-antigen, these cells could be removed by using specific monoclonal antibodies. In practice, it would be impossible to raise a monoclonal antibody for each individual patient requiring treatment. Fortunately, TCR genes can be divided into different families based on sequence homology. Various monoclonal antibodies are available which recognize all gene products belonging to the same family. Thus if a 'disease-associated' TCR can be located to a particular Vβ family, a viable alternative treatment may be the use of Vβ family-specific antibodies. Such antibodies would remove all T cells expressing rearrangements of genes in this family but leave T cells utilizing other Vβ gene families unaffected.

In summary, immunotherapy offers an exciting future for the treatment of ADs if the problem of non-specific suppression can be overcome.

7.8 Conclusions

The prognosis of AD is variable. Some are life-threatening, others of little consequence in terms of life expectancy. The majority shorten life to some extent. Chronic AD may be complicated by malignant transformation. Tumors of the immune system are the most common type of malignancy.

Treatment of AD falls into four categories. Specific replacement therapy may be given to patients with malfunctioning organs. Disease modifying therapy is used in RA, SLE and dermatitis herpetiformis. In those ADs with serious morbidity immunosuppressive therapy may be used. This may consist of corticosteroids or cytotoxic drugs. Alternatively, the patient may be physically depleted of lymphocytes.

There are a number of experimental forms of immunotherapy, rational drug design, T cell vaccination, orally induced tolerance and T cell monoclonal antibodies. Whilst none is yet of proven clinical value, these developments are likely to lead to a major therapeutic breakthrough.

Further reading

Adorini, L. and Nagy, Z.A. (1990) Peptide competition for antigen presentation. *Immunol. Today*, **11**, 21.

Cohen, I. (1986) Regulation of autoimmune disease; physiological and therapeutic. *Immunol. Rev.*, **94**, 5.

Dawes, P.T. and Symmons, D.P.M. (1992) Short term effects of anti-rheumatic drugs. *Clinics in Rheumatol. Dis.* **6** (1).

Lohse, A.W. and Cohen, I.R. (1990) Mechanisms of resistance to autoimmune disease induced by T cell vaccination. in *The Molecular Biology of Autoimmune Disease*. (A.G. Demaine, J.P. Banga, A.M. McGregor, eds). Nato ASI series H, Cell Biology, Volume **38**. Springer-Verlag, Berlin, p. 333.

Panayi, G.S., Lanchbury, J.S.S. and Kingsley, G. (1991) First International symposium of the immunotherapy of the rheumatic diseases. *Br. J. Rheumatol.*, Suppl. **30**.

Thompson, H.S.G. and Staines, N.A. (1991) Could specific oral tolerance be a therapy for autoimmune disease? *Immunol. Today*, **11**, 396.

8
EPILOG

In the preceding chapters we have attempted to cover the clinical conditions loosely grouped together as ADs; to describe some of the immunological, genetic and environmental threads they have in common; and to put them into the context of current thinking.

AD is the end result of a number of different but interconnecting components, each providing an important contribution to overall disease susceptibility, although the additive effect of such factors may be crucial. AD has frequently been described as having a polygenic basis which has been superimposed on to a major environmental background. Such complex inter-relationships provoked us, in 1986, to suggest the analogy of a jigsaw puzzle in which the overall picture only emerges as the various key pieces slot together. Needless to say many pieces are yet to be found, and of those that

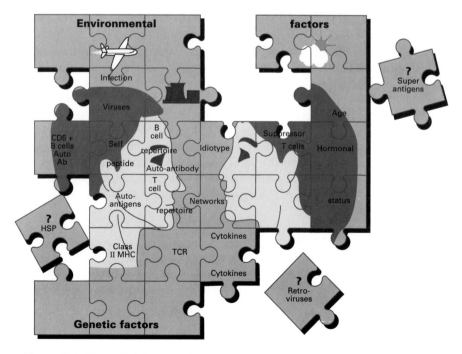

Figure 8.1: The unfinished puzzle.

we assume fit together, some may belong to a different puzzle (*Figure 8.1*). Likewise, Schonfeld and Isenberg view autoimmunity as a mosaic of interconnecting pieces where different components and processes relate to each other.

The failure to identify the main environmental factors in ADs remains a major deficiency in our understanding. The study of varying disease expression and frequency in different races, climates, geographical and environmental settings continues to yield clues as to possible triggers for AD processes. New technological advances which enable minute traces of viral DNA to be detected may provide some answers. Similarly, new methods have ensured that characterization of auto-antigens continues at a steady pace, although why auto-antigens should become self-immunogenic remains unclear.

Serious deficiencies also lie in our understanding of the genetic basis for the development of autoimmunity. A major advance came from demonstrating HLA associations with ADs and a biological basis in terms of antigen presentation and MHC restriction has become apparent. In addition it is now known that MHC background influences the final composition of the TCR repertoire. For most diseases, it is estimated that HLA accounts for 50%, at the most, of the genetic component. Our obsession with the HLA complex may have delayed interest in looking elsewhere in the genome. Such studies have become a realistic proposition as a result of recent advances in molecular biology.

The innovation of the polymerase chain reaction (PCR) has enabled the characterization of disease susceptibility genes. Using sense and antisense synthetic oligonucleotide primers, specific short regions of DNA are rapidly amplified in an exponential replication of the original sequence. A powerful modification of this technique is 'anchored PCR', which can be used to amplify stretches of DNA away from a known reference sequence. These techniques are now being used in the characterization of TCR and immunoglobulin variable region genes and to determine which idiotypic rearrangements are implicated in recognition of auto-antigens. PCR has many more applications which are being introduced for the potential analysis of disease susceptibility genes. The Human Genome Project will have implications for the identification and characterization of disease susceptibility genes. One area of great potential is the use of microsatellite sequences of repeat DNA bases. These include $(CA)_n$ repeats (where n is 10–60) which are evenly distributed throughout the human genome (approximately every 50 kb), TCTG repeats and variable poly(A) tracts of *Alu*I sequences. More than 10% of microsatellite sequences are highly polymorphic and probes used to detect these polymorphisms can be utilized in linkage studies of ADs in multiplex families.

Physical mapping of chromosomes requires the cloning of DNA. Until now the largest inserts of DNA (35–45 kb) have been cloned in cosmid vectors. A recent advance has been the construction of DNA libraries in yeast cells, known as yeast artificial chromosomes (YACs). Typical YACs contain single fragments of DNA that are up to two megabases in size and are stable during growth. YAC libraries provide, for the first time, a realistic means to search at specific sites in the human genome for informative microsatellite DNA probes which will help identify linkage between chromosomal areas and AD.

A central tenet in immunology has been that self-tolerance is due to clonal deletion and anergy, brought about by negative selection of T cells in the thymus and mechanisms for peripheral tolerance. The 'Holy Grail' for immunologists interested in autoimmunity is how these mechanisms of tolerance are avoided or deficient for particular self-antigens. Healthy individuals appear to have lymphocytes capable of recognizing self-antigens and so limited autoimmunity may be the rule rather than the exception. An important consideration is, therefore, whether all autoimmune processes are harmful and at what point we classify these processes as diseases. We have perhaps all been guilty of believing too readily the dogma of 'horror autotoxicus' and accepting that self-recognition and response is the ultimate immunological sin.

An increasingly popular school of thought, championed by Irun Cohen, is that self-recognition to a limited and controlled degree is an important adjunct to the immune response to foreign antigens. This concept argues that only a restricted number of dominant auto-antigens exists, many of which are key functional molecules and conserved in most life forms. The best examples may be HSPs and DNA. Varying degrees of sequence homology exist between self-like microbial molecules and auto-antigens, which presents something of a paradox. Cohen suggests that relatively large numbers of B cells (mainly CD5-positive) are capable of recognizing these conserved 'self-like' antigens and provide an important amplification system where non-conserved, microbial-specific antigens within the same molecule can readily be presented to T cells. It is suggested that T cells capable of recognizing conserved 'self-like' antigens also exist. These self-epitopes can function as carriers for responses to other epitopes and thus provide an important source of ready-made T cell help. The control of such 'auto-reactive' B and T cells is invested in idiotypic networks which operate to check progressive autoimmunity. However, the recognition of non-conserved antigens coupled to self-antigen will trigger a protective aggressive response.

The potential for recognizing a limited series of dominant auto-antigens may therefore be pre-programmed together with the initiation of controlling idiotypic networks for these antigens. It is suggested that the body uses such cellular idiotypic networks to produce an immunological reference picture and representation of what is self – what has been termed the immunological homunculus ('little man') by Cohen.

Following on from this concept, the onset of AD is seen as occurring when the controlling regulatory networks go awry and when the response to self-antigen becomes a progressive and pathogenic process. This attractive idea is compatible both with the increasing prevalence of autoimmune conditions with age and with the relapsing/remitting course of many conditions.

The study of autoimmunity requires the basic scientist and the clinician to work in close collaboration: only in that way will relevant and rapid progress be made. A good example of such collaboration is found in the field of pediatric rheumatology. Clinicians treating children with juvenile chronic arthritis observed that there seemed to be three distinct groups based on their long-term outcome: children with so-called pauciarticular arthritis (four or fewer joints involved at the onset), those with polyarticular arthritis (five or more joints involved at onset) and those with systemic onset (fever and rash at the onset). These groups vary in terms of the mean age at onset, the relative proportion of girls and boys affected as well as the long-term prognosis. Children with pauciarticular arthritis often have eye involvement, a relatively rare complication in the other two groups. The immunologist has demonstrated that this eye involvement is usually associated with ANA positivity. ANA thus becomes a useful screening test for identifying those at risk of eye problems. Molecular biologists have also shown recently that these groups of children are genetically distinct from one another in terms of their HLA.

In other situations it may be the basic scientist who identifies an unusual haplotype or antibody in some individuals out of a group of patients thought to have homogeneous disease. Thus anti-Ro antibodies in SLE are found to identify patients with photosensitive rashes. To return to the analogy of the jigsaw puzzle it may be said that the clinician has the lid of the box showing the finished picture and the basic scientist holds the pieces, some of which belong to a different puzzle. By working together the puzzle will be completed more quickly.

Further reading

Cohen, I.R. and Young, D.B. (1991) Autoimmunity, microbial immunity and the immunological homunculus. *Immunol. Today*, **12**, 105.

Schlessinger, D. (1990) Yeast artificial chromosomes: tools for mapping and analysis of complex genomes. *Trends Genetics*, **6**, 254.

Todd, J.A., Aitman, T.J., Cornall, R.J. *et al.* (1991). Genetic analysis of autoimmune type I diabetes mellitus in mice. *Nature*, **351**, 542.

Weber, J.L. (1990) Informativeness of human $(dC-dA)_n \bullet (dG-dT)_n$ polymorphisms. *Genomics*, **7**, 524.

Weber, J.L. and May, P.E., (1989) Abundant classes of human DNA polymorphisms which can be typed using polymerase chain reaction. *Am. J. Hum. Genet.*, **44**, 388.

APPENDIX A. GLOSSARY

Adjuvant: an agent administered with an antigen which induces heightened immune responses.

Affinity chromatography: column chromatography in which the support medium is bound chemically to a specific antibody. The complementary antigen can be purified through its binding to the antibody and subsequently eluted. Alternatively, antibodies can be purified by the attachment of specific antigen to the column.

Alleles: alternative forms of a gene occurring at the same position (locus) on a chromosome.

Allotypic variation: variation between individuals of the same species.

Apoptosis: self destruction of cells in a programmed way.

Autoradiography: the location of molecules or antigens by a method using radiolabeled probes and photographic film.

Bursa of Fabricius: lymphoid tissue, important in the maturation of B lymphocytes, which is found in birds.

cDNA library: a method whereby cDNA can be cloned into bacterial cells and screened.

Cirrhosis: a fibrotic condition affecting the liver.

Cis: genes inherited together on the same chromosome.

Complement pathway: an enzyme cascade system which is activated when certain classes of antibody recognize and bind cell surface antigen. Activated complement can lyse cells.

Disease concordance: the proportion of identical twin pairs in which both twins have the same disease.

Disease incidence: the number of new cases of the disease in a given population which develop during a specified time period.

Disease prevalence: the number of individuals in a given population who have the disease at a particular point in time.

Dizygotic twins: twins derived from two different fertilized eggs.

DNA – cDNA: complementary DNA made by the enzyme reverse transcriptase using mRNA as a template.

DNA – germline: total DNA genome derived from a fertilized egg and passed on to each cell through mitosis.

DNA polymerase: an enzyme which synthesizes double-stranded DNA from single-stranded DNA.

DNA sequence homology: the degree of identity between gene sequences.

Efficacy: how well a drug or treatment works.

ELISA: enzyme-linked immunosorbent assay. Methods using enzyme-conjugated species-specific antibodies as probes to detect the binding of test antibodies to antigen. The binding of antibody is quantified by the degree of enzyme-dependent color development of a substrate.

Emphysema: a chronic lung disease associated with over-distension of the lungs.

Epitope: the part of an antigen which is recognized by and combines with either an antibody molecule or a T cell receptor.

Epitope-discontinuous: epitope determined by the three-dimensional folding of the antigen molecule.

Epitope-linear: epitope determined by a continuous linear sequence of amino acid residues.

Epitope-mapping: method by which epitopes recognized by T or B cells can be determined.

Epitope-shared: a sequence recognized by antibodies or T cells which is common to more than one protein.

Eukaryotic DNA: DNA from the cells of higher organisms which have a discernable nucleus.

Expression vector: a cloning vector which will enable foreign gene to be expressed in the host organism.

Flow cytometry: a procedure in which cells or particles are labeled with a fluorochrome, either directly or using conjugated antibody, and passed individually through a laser beam. The light emitted from each particle is measured and analyzed to gather information regarding the proportion of cells possessing a particular antigen. Information on cell size and antigen density can also be obtained.

Gag protein: typical retroviruses have a gag gene encoding a precursor polyprotein which is cleaved to yield the capsid proteins

Gene: sequence of nucleotides in the DNA which encodes a single polypeptide. Genes contain both exons (coding sequences) and introns (non-coding sequences).

Gene – deletion: a process whereby a gene or parts of a gene are deleted in order to investigate the effects in the expressed product.

Gene – disease susceptibility: a gene thought to be responsible for allowing an individual to develop a particular disease.

Gene – exons: nucleotide sequences of a gene which encode for the expressed product.

Gene – introns: nucleotide sequences of a gene which do not encode for expressed product.

Gene linkage: inheritance of two or more genes as a single unit as a result of their close proximity on the chromosome.

Gene mutation: event or process whereby the nucleotide sequence of a gene is changed. This may occur 'naturally' in a random manner as a result of chemical, irradiation or other environmental effects. Alternatively, it can be engineered specifically by methods such as site-directed mutagenesis.

Gene splicing: methods by which nucleotide sequences from different genes are brought together to produce a new gene.

Gene – transfection: methods in which a new or 'foreign' gene is introduced into the genome of a cell.

Genotype: the genetic characteristics of an individual.

Germinal centers: areas of active lymphocyte cell division within lymphoid tissues.

Glycosylation: the addition of carbohydrate to proteins.

Graft-versus-host disease: a condition which can occur when an immunocompetent graft (e.g. bone marrow cells) is given to a largely immunologically incompetent host (irradiated recipient). If the donor and recipient are not identically matched the graft can start to reject the host.

Granulocytes: neutrophil, basophil or eosinophil white blood cells.

Granuloma (plural granulomata): a small mass of granulation tissue.

Haplotype: combination of alleles of linked genes inherited 'en bloc' on the same chromosome.

Heat shock proteins: proteins originally through to be produced by cells as a response to stress. It is now known that they are made by cells under normal physiological conditions.

Hemopoiesis: the generation of blood cells from bone marrow stem cells.

Heterozygous: the possession by an individual of two different alleles at the same locus on each of a pair of chromosomes.

Hirsutism: abnormal hairiness.

Homeostasis: the dynamic process by which a stable equilibrium of tissue chemistry is maintained.

Hydrophobicity profile: profile reflecting the distribution of hydrophilic or hydrophobic amino acid residues in a protein. This profile can be used to predict which residues are likely to be exposed on the surface of a molecule and contribute to its antigenicity.

Hypergammaglobulinemia: abnormally high circulating levels of immunoglobulins.

Hypervariable regions: regions within proteins such as immunoglobulins, histocompatibility antigens and T cell receptors where the majority of sequence variation exists.

Hypothalamus: an organ in the brain which governs the functioning of all the endocrine glands in the body.

Idiotype: the antigen combining sites of antibody molecules which have unique specificity for a antigen. These are encoded by variable light and heavy immunoglobulin genes.

Idiotypic network: a regulatory network proposed by Jerne where the idiotypic specificity of one antibody molecule provides the antigen for another antibody which in turn provides the antigen for another and so on. The effect of producing such idiotypic antibodies is to switch off and regulate antibody producing clones.

Immune complex: the combination of antigen and antibody in varying proportions. Depending on the size of complex formed it can be soluble or precipitated.

Immune surveillance: a mechanism whereby the immune response constantly maintains the integrity of the body by detecting and eliminating malignant and foreign cells which do not measure up to the strict definition of what is self.

Immunoglobulin class switching: a process whereby immunoglobulins change from having one type of constant heavy chain to another.

Indirect immunofluorescence: a method of detecting auto-antibodies or auto-antigens through the use of microscopy and anti-species specific antibodies conjugated with dyes which fluoresce in ultraviolet radiation.

In-situ **hybridization:** binding of a labeled cloned gene or oligonucleotide probe to a large DNA molecule, usually a chromosome. This technique can be used for gene mapping.

Intergrins: a family of cell surface adhesion molecules.

Interleukins: cytokines produced by a variety of cell types which regulate many immune functions as well as other processes.

Iso-electric focusing: separation of proteins on a pH gradient by electrophoresis. Proteins migrate to their isoelectric point.

Linkage disequilibrium: occurs when the alleles of two linked genes are observed together at a higher frequency than would be predicted from their individual gene frequencies.

Lymphokine: cytokine produced by cells of the immune system.

Lymphoma: a solid tumor resulting from malignant transformation in lymphoid tissue.

Lymphopenia: abnormally low circulating lymphocyte count.

Lymphotropic virus: a virus which specifically or preferentially infects lymphocytes.

Macrophage: phagocytic cells derived from monocytes which are capable of ingesting foreign cells and particles and, after protein degradation, presenting them to T lymphocytes.

Major histocompatibility complex: a family of highly polymorphic genes encoding a variety of cell surface glycoprotein transplantation antigens which are responsible for the presentation of peptide antigens to T lymphocytes. They provide the mechanism by which self can be distinguished from non-self.

Mast cells: cells containing a variety of inflammatory substances (such as vasoactive amines, histamine and heparin) which can be released through the action of IgE antibodies.

Megaloblastic anemia: an anemia in which the precursor red blood cells in the bone marrow are abnormally large.

Menarche: the time of onset of menstruation.

Microsatellite sequences: small repetitive sequences of DNA bases in the genome. These can be very polymorphic.

Mitogen: an agent which induces cells non-specifically to enter mitosis and proliferate.

Mixed lymphocyte culture: an *in-vitro* culture of lymphocytes from two individuals. The degree of lymphoproliferation indicates the level of difference between MHC antigen profile.

Monoclonal antibody: antibody produced by a hybrid cell which has been made by fusing a stimulated B lymphocyte with a myeloma cell line. The fused 'hybridoma' cell is manipulated to be clonal and thus antibody with a single isotype and a single specificity is produced. The hybridoma is immortal and can be kept in continuous culture to produce limitless supplies of identical antibody.

Monozygotic twins: identical twins derived from the same fertilized egg.

Myeloma: a malignant B cell/plasma cell tumor which will continue to divide clonally and produce vast quantities of antibody of monoclonal specificity.

Narcolepsy: condition where the patient has uncontrolled bouts of falling asleep.

Non-Hodgkins lymphoma: a family of malignant tumors developing from lymphoid tissue. They may be of B cell or T cell origin.

Nucleotide triphosphates: the basic 'building blocks' needed to synthesize DNA molecules. These are deoxyadenosine triphosphate (dATP), deoxyguanosine triphosphate (dGTP), deoxycytidine triphosphate (dCTP) and deoxythymidine triphosphate (dTTP).

Oligonucleotide probes: preparations of synthetic oligonucleotides, designed to hybridize with specific DNA sequences.

Ophthalmitis: inflammation of the whole eye.

Oral tolerance: induction of tolerance to a foreign antigen by repeated oral administration of the antigen.

Orchitis: inflammation of the male gonads.

Paraprotein: the immunoglobulin produced in very high concentrations in myeloma.

Parenteral: administration of a drug or other substance by a non-oral route.

Parotid gland: one of the salivary glands situated just in front of the ear.

PCR (polymerase chain reaction): a method in which a single gene copy is amplified specifically and exponentially, using oligonucleotide primers and DNA polymerase.

Penetrance: frequency of the phenotypic expression of a gene in affected individuals. Penetrance can be complete, where every individual carrying the gene will be affected, or incomplete, where some individuals may carry the gene but not manifest the disease (phenotype).

Phenotype: the observed characteristics of an individual.

Plasma cells: end-stage differentiated B lymphocytes whose sole role is to secrete large quantities of antibody.

Polygenic disease: a disease caused by the inheritance and action of more than one gene.

Polymorphism: two or more different alleles in a population, each of which is present at a frequency higher than that expected by mutation.

Prokaryotic DNA: DNA from elementary life forms such as bacteria which have no discernable nuclear membrane.

Pseudogene: a gene which cannot give rise to a functional product because of one or more mutational changes in its sequence.

Puerperium: the few weeks following the delivery of an infant (the term refers to the mother).

Pulmonary: relating to the lung.

Recombinant antigen: antigen produced through recombinant DNA technology. The gene responsible for the antigen is manipulated into bacterial cells which synthesize large quantities of the antigen.

Recombination distance: a measure of distance between linked genes calculated by examining the number of cross-over events between the genes during meiosis.

Restriction enzyme: an enzyme, derived from bacteria which has the ability to digest and thus cleave DNA at particular nucleotide sequences. This can be used as the basis for the detection of gene polymorphisms as the band sizes of DNA fragments can vary for different alleles (restriction fragment length polymorphism). These are visualized on Southern blots using labeled gene-specific probes.

Retroviruses: RNA viruses which utilize reverse transcriptase for replication and to integrate into DNA of cells.

Reverse transcriptase: enzyme which produces a DNA sequence from an RNA template.

Rheumatoid factors: auto-antibodies made to the Fc component of immunoglobulin molecules. Rheumatoid factors are usually of the IgM class but can also be IgG or IgA classes.

Somatic mutation: a mutation which occurs at the individual cell level and will thus not be inherited through germline DNA.

Splenectomy: removal of the spleen.

Stem cells: precursor cells which proliferate and give rise to more differentiated cells.

Superantigens: antigens which can activate large proportions of the T cell repertoire through their ability to form ligands between class II molecules and Vβ elements of T cell receptors.

Supratype: a haplotypic combination of alleles which has been 'held together' and conserved through linkage disequilibrium.

Synovitis: inflammation of the joint lining.

T cell – helper: CD4-positive antigen cell which is important in both B and T cell responses.

T cell receptor: receptor present on the surface of T cells, capable of recognizing and combining with antigens presented in the context of MHC molecules. Two types of TCR exist, one comprising α/β chains, the other γ/δ chains.

T cell repertoire: the total available range of antigens which can be recognized by T cells in an individual.

T cell – suppressor: CD8-positive antigen T lymphocyte capable of modulating immune responses by suppressing other T cells.

T cell vaccination: the switching off of specific immune responses by 'vaccination' with treated T cells specific for the relevant antigen.

Thrombocytopenia: abnormally low numbers of platelets in the peripheral blood.

Thyroiditis: inflammation of the thyroid gland.

***Trans*:** Genes that are not on the same chromosome.

Transgenic mice: a strain of mice in which a non-mouse gene (usually human) has been introduced into the germline DNA.

Vasculitis: inflammation of blood vessels.

Vector: DNA capable of replication in a host organism, into which a gene can be inserted to form a recombinant DNA molecule.

Waldenströms macroglobulinemia: a malignant condition of IgM producing B cells.

Western blotting: a procedure in which antibodies are used as 'probes' to detect proteins which have been separated electrophoretically under reducing or non-reducing conditions and blotted on to membrane. Bands of immunoprecipitation can be detected by autoradiography or ELISA techniques.

X-ray crystallography: by manipulation of conditions, crystals of pure protein can be grown. When subjected to X-ray diffraction studies considerable information relating to the three-dimensional structure of the molecule can be gained.

Yeast artificial chromosomes: yeast chromosomes that are created when large inserts of DNA (usually human) are cloned into the DNA of yeast cells.

INDEX